complete guide
to CARB COUNTING
4th Edition

Practical Tools for Better Diabetes Meal Planning

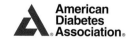

American
Diabetes
Association.

Associate Publisher, Books, Abe Ogden; *Director, Book Operations*, Victor Van Beuren; *Managing Editor, Books*, John Clark; *Associate Director, Book Marketing*, Annette Reape; *Acquisitions Editor*, Jaclyn Konich; *Senior Manager, Book Editing*, Lauren Wilson; *Project Manager*, Wendy Martin-Shuma; *Writer*, Jennifer Arnold; *Composition*, Circle Graphics; *Cover Design*, Jenn French Designs; *Printer*, Versa Press.

Printed in the United States of America

1 3 5 7 9 10 8 6 4 2

The suggestions and information contained in this publication are generally consistent with the *Standards of Medical Care in Diabetes* and other policies of the American Diabetes Association, but they do not represent the policy or position of the Association or any of its boards or committees. Reasonable steps have been taken to ensure the accuracy of the information presented. However, the American Diabetes Association cannot ensure the safety or efficacy of any product or service described in this publication. Individuals are advised to consult a physician or other appropriate health care professional before undertaking any diet or exercise program or taking any medication referred to in this publication. Professionals must use and apply their own professional judgment, experience, and training and should not rely solely on the information contained in this publication before prescribing any diet, exercise, or medication. The American Diabetes Association—its officers, directors, employees, volunteers, and members—assumes no responsibility or liability for personal or other injury, loss, or damage that may result from the suggestions or information in this publication.

Sacha Uelmen conducted the internal review of this book to ensure that it meets American Diabetes Association guidelines.

@ The paper in this publication meets the requirements of the ANSI Standard Z39.48-1992 (permanence of paper).

ADA titles may be purchased for business or promotional use or for special sales. To purchase more than 50 copies of this book at a discount, or for custom editions of this book with your logo, contact the American Diabetes Association at the address below or at booksales@diabetes.org.

American Diabetes Association
2451 Crystal Drive, Suite 900
Arlington, VA 22202

DOI: 10.2337/ 9781580406840

Library of Congress Cataloging-in-Publication Data

Names: American Diabetes Association, issuing body.
Title: The complete guide to carb counting : practical tools for better
diabetes meal planning / American Diabetes Association.
Description: 4th edition. | Arlington : American Diabetes Association, [2019]
| Revision of: Complete guide to carb counting / Hope S. Warshaw, Karmeen
Kulkarni. 2011. 3rd ed. | Includes bibliographical references and index.
Identifiers: LCCN 2018039971 | ISBN 9781580406840 (pbk. : alk. paper)
Subjects: LCSH: Diabetes—Diet therapy. | Food—Carbohydrate content.
Classification: LCC RC662 .W313 2019 | DDC 616.4/620654—dc23
LC record available at https://lccn.loc.gov/2018039971

Table of Contents

Previous Editions

The Complete Guide to Carb Counting, 1st edition (2001)
Hope S. Warshaw, MMSc, RD, CDE, and Karmeen Kulkarni, MS, RD, CDE

The Complete Guide to Carb Counting, 2nd edition (2004)
Hope S. Warshaw, MMSc, RD, CDE, and Karmeen Kulkarni, MS, RD, CDE

The Complete Guide to Carb Counting, 3rd edition (2011)
Hope S. Warshaw, MMSc, RD, CDE, BC-ADM, and
Karmeen Kulkari, MS, RD, CDE, BC-ADM, with Jennifer Arnold

What Is Carb Counting?

In this chapter, you'll learn:

- Basic facts about carbohydrate
- How carbohydrate affects blood glucose
- How carb counting works for blood glucose management

Carb counting is a meal-planning method that can help people with diabetes manage their blood glucose levels. It can work for people with type 1 or type 2 diabetes and can be adapted to the unique needs of each person. Carb counting works along with other elements of a diabetes care plan, such as medications and physical activity, to help you feel your best now and for years to come.

Is carb counting right for you? Only you can answer that question. We hope this book will help you learn more about what carb counting is and how it works. Then, with input from your diabetes care team, you can decide if it could work for you. Throughout the book, you'll find step-by-step directions on how to use carb counting and some self-assessment tools to help you decide if carb counting is right for you.

What Is Carbohydrate, Anyway?

Carbohydrate is a type of nutrient found in certain foods and beverages. Other nutrients include protein, fat, vitamins, and minerals. Each nutrient has an important role to play in the body. Carbohydrate's job is to provide cells with the energy they need to grow and function.

When you eat carbohydrate, your body breaks it down into glucose (the scientific name for a type of sugar) and releases that glucose into your bloodstream. But glucose can't get to hungry cells on its own. It needs the hormone insulin to show it the way. Insulin works sort of like a guide or a chaperone, leading the glucose to cells that need fuel. So you see, carbohydrates are not "bad"—in fact, they are essential to good health.

Why Count Carbs?

As we explained above, the body breaks down carbohydrate into glucose. Insulin then helps move the glucose to hungry cells that need the glucose for fuel.

In people with diabetes, that process doesn't work correctly. With type 1 diabetes, the body does not produce insulin at all. In type 2 diabetes, the body does not produce enough insulin, or is not able to use insulin effectively to move the glucose in the bloodstream to the cells. That is why people with diabetes have high levels of glucose in their bloodstreams.

Carb counting—tracking the amount of carbohydrate you eat for meals and snacks—can help you predict how much glucose will be entering your bloodstream after you eat. If you have prediabetes or type 2 diabetes, carb counting can help you manage your blood glucose level and feel your best, whether or not you take any diabetes medications. If you have type 1 diabetes, carb counting can help you match your mealtime insulin dosage to the amount of carbs you are eating.

A Note for People with Type 1 Diabetes

Using carb counting to determine insulin doses is an advanced skill, covered in more detail in Chapter 11. The rest of the chapters in this book will give you a good foundation on the principles of carb counting so you'll be ready when you get to that chapter.

Which Foods Contain Carbohydrate?

When you hear "carbs," you may think of breads, pasta, and rice. And you're right—those foods do contain carbohydrate. But they're not the only ones. Here's a more complete list of foods that contain carbohydrate:

- Grains like rice, oatmeal, and barley
- Grain-based foods like bread, cereal, pasta, and crackers

- Starchy vegetables like potatoes, peas, and corn
- Fruit and fruit juice
- Milk and yogurt
- Beans like pinto beans, black beans, and kidney beans
- Soy products like veggie burgers and tofu
- Sweets and snacks like sodas, juice drinks, cake, cookies, candy, and chips

Nonstarchy vegetables like lettuce, cucumbers, broccoli, and cauliflower also contain carbohydrate, but in such small amounts that they do not affect blood glucose. (See Appendix 1 under Vegetables to compare the carb count differences between starchy and nonstarchy vegetables.)

After reading this list, you might wonder which foods do *not* contain carbohydrate. Generally, proteins (beef, poultry, pork, seafood, and eggs) and fats (oil, butter, and nuts) do not contain carbs.

A Note about Proteins and Fats

Although proteins and fats aren't part of daily carb counting totals, carb counters still need to pay attention to them. They contain calories and other nutrients that are also important to a healthy eating plan. You will learn more about protein and fats and how they affect eating plans in Chapter 6.

How Much Carbohydrate Is in Certain Foods?

As you may guess from the name, carb counting involves adding up all the carbohydrate in the foods you eat. To do that, of course, you need to know *how much* carbohydrate is in different foods. You'll soon learn that there can be a wide range in the amount of carbs in different foods, even within the same food group.

Take a look at Table 1.1. As you can see, a medium banana has 27 grams of carbohydrate, while 1 cup of strawberries has 11 grams of carbohydrate. Both are fruits, but the banana has more than twice the amount of carbohydrate. The same goes in the starchy vegetable group—a large baked potato has more than twice the grams of carbohydrate as 1 cup of green peas.

Table 1.1 Grams of Carbohydrate in Different Types of Food

	Serving size	Grams of carbohydrate
FRUITS		
Banana	1 medium	27
Strawberries	1 cup	11
Watermelon	1 cup	7.5
STARCHY VEGETABLES		
White potato	1 large, baked	63
Butternut squash	1 cup, cooked cubes	21.5
Green peas	1 cup, cooked	25
BREADS AND GRAINS		
Bagel	1 plain (100 g)	51.8
Brown rice, medium grain	1 cup, cooked	45.8
Flour tortilla, 6-inch	1 tortilla	15
Spaghetti	1 cup, cooked	43
DAIRY PRODUCTS		
Fruit yogurt, low-fat	1 8-oz container	42
Milk, 2%	1 cup	11
SUGARY DRINKS		
Cola	12 oz	38
Ginger ale	12 oz	32
Sports drink	1 bottle (about 20.5 fluid oz)	39

For more information, see *Choose Your Foods: Food Lists for Diabetes*, a booklet from the Academy of Nutrition and Dietetics and American Diabetes Association.

If you decide to try carb counting, you'll rely on charts and tools like this to track the amount of carbohydrate you eat throughout the day. Throughout this book, we'll share resources to help you.

Are All Carbohydrates the Same?

The answer is yes and no. Scientists now understand that all carbohydrates affect blood glucose in the same way. That means that once carbohydrate is broken down into glucose, the body doesn't know whether that glucose came from a banana or a donut. All carbohydrate, no matter the food source, is broken down into glucose that enters the bloodstream in the same way. So when you're practicing carb counting, all carbohydrate is counted the same way.

However, there *are* different kinds of carbohydrate in our food. In general, there are three kinds of carbohydrate: starches, sugars, and fiber. You'll see them listed on food labels (you'll learn more about food labels in Chapter 3) and referred to in books and articles about healthy eating. While all three affect blood glucose in the same way, they each have unique effects on other aspects of our health. Let's look at each one separately.

Starches

Starch is sometimes referred to as a complex carbohydrate. Complex carbohydrates include beans and lentils; grains like oats, barley, and rice; and certain vegetables. You'll often hear diabetes care professionals refer to "starchy vegetables" and "nonstarchy vegetables." Some vegetables, such as peas, corn, and potatoes, have much more starch and therefore many more grams of carbohydrate. See Appendix 1 under Vegetables to compare the carb count differences between starchy and nonstarchy vegetables.

Sugars

There are many different kinds of sugar and many different sources. The most obvious probably is the granulated sugar and brown sugar used in baking and cooking. There are also many kinds of sugar added to processed foods. (Sometimes you'll see these types of sugar listed on food labels as "added sugars.") Then there are the sugars that occur naturally in foods, like fructose in fruit and lactose in milk.

For many years, people with diabetes were told to avoid sugar. But now we know that *all* types of carbohydrate affect blood glucose in the same way and that the *total* amount of carbohydrate in a food or meal is the most important factor. As we go on, we'll learn more about how to manage sugars as part of your eating plan.

Can I Eat Sweets While Managing My Blood Glucose?

The short answer is yes. As long as you account for the carbohydrate in your eating plan (and adjust your diabetes medications, if you take them), sugary foods and sweets can be worked into your blood glucose management plan. Carb counting can help you do this, and you'll learn how in this book.

This doesn't mean that it is healthful to regularly eat candy, cake, and cookies. That isn't healthful for anyone! Realize that even a small serving of these types of foods contains a lot of carbohydrate. These foods also typically contain a lot of calories and fat. So you'll want to limit them to special occasions and choose small portions.

....

Fiber

As with sugar, there are many different types of fiber in our foods. Fiber is found in whole, unprocessed foods like whole fruits and vegetables, raw nuts and seeds, and beans. Fiber is an essential part of a healthy eating plan for *all* people, not just people with diabetes. Healthy amounts of fiber in our diets help protect our hearts from disease and keep our digestive systems working well. Some fibers are also helpful in weight loss because they make you feel full and satisfied.

Why Is It Important to Manage Blood Glucose Levels?

Keeping your blood glucose levels within your target range helps you feel your best. Keeping levels in target is also the best way to prevent or delay complications of diabetes, such as heart, eye, and kidney problems.

Table 1.2 shows the American Diabetes Association recommended target ranges for three different tests used to assess blood glucose levels. These are general guidelines for the "average" person—each person's target levels will be different, based on age,

Table 1.2 American Diabetes Association Target Ranges for Blood Glucose and A1C Levels*

Test	Goal
Average fasting and premeal blood glucose	80–130 mg/dL
Average postmeal blood glucose level (1–2 hours after the start of a meal)	<180 mg/dL
A1C (%)	<7% (normal range is based on 4–6%)

*Or glucose level/A1C recommended by your health care provider. For more information, visit www.diabetes.org.

other health conditions you have, how long you have had diabetes, and other factors. You and your diabetes care team will work together to set blood glucose targets that make sense for you.

People who are newly diagnosed with diabetes often have blood glucose levels outside the target range. With the help of their diabetes care team, newly diagnosed people learn to manage their diabetes through tracking their food, activity, and medications and learning how each affects their blood glucose levels. Carb counting is one tool that can help.

Keeping your blood glucose levels within your target range helps you feel your best. Keeping levels in target is also the best way to prevent or delay complications of diabetes, such as heart, eye, and kidney problems.

Is Carb Counting the Same as a Low-Carb Diet?

The short answer is no. There are many different variations of low-carb weight loss plans, but in general, they call for restricting carbohydrates dramatically, to far lower levels than the American Diabetes Association recommends. Many diabetes experts say that there is not enough evidence to recommend low-carb diets, especially to people with type 2 diabetes. There is just not enough proof that they work and are safe in the long term.

If you are trying to lose weight, it is most important to consider the total number of calories you eat every day. Healthy carbohydrate sources like fruits, vegetables,

A healthy eating plan for people with diabetes is generally the same as a healthy eating plan for anyone else: a varied diet low in saturated and trans fats, moderate in salt and sugar, with meals based on lean protein, nonstarchy vegetables, whole grains, healthy fats, and fruit.

whole grains, and low-fat dairy foods are an important part of your daily calorie intake. You *do* want to limit the not-so-healthy carbohydrate sources, like foods that contain added sugars, because they contribute concentrated amounts of calories and fats and add little in the way of essential vitamins and minerals.

The reality is, a healthy eating plan for people with diabetes is generally the same as a healthy eating plan for anyone else: a varied diet low in saturated and trans fats, moderate in salt and sugar, with meals based on lean protein, nonstarchy vegetables, whole grains, healthy fats, and fruit. There is no ideal percentage of calories from carbohydrate, protein, and fat for all people with diabetes. Each person's eating plan should be based on their preferences, patterns, and health goals.

How Does Carb Counting Work?

OK, let's get to it—how exactly do you do this? Here are the basics:

- You and your diabetes care provider will set a goal for the amount of carbs you should eat for each meal and snack throughout the day.
- You will use a variety of tools to choose foods that help you stay within those goals.
- If you're using a blood glucose meter, you will watch to see how your carb intake affects your blood glucose levels and make changes as needed.

That's it! We'll explain each of those bullet points in detail in the next three chapters and give you opportunities to practice with real-life examples. You'll learn:

- How to find carb count information about the foods and beverages you consume

- How to measure the ingredients and portions of the foods you eat
- How to keep track of what you eat and the amount of carbs in your meals

After you learn these basics, the remaining chapters will build on that foundation with more information about other nutrients in your foods, how to navigate recipes and restaurant meals, how carb counting works with diabetes medications, and some more advanced concepts. Let's get started!

Let's Review

See if you can answer these questions. Refer back to the chapter if you need help.

- What is carbohydrate? What is its job in the body? *A type of nutrient; provides energy for cells*
- How does carb counting help with blood glucose management? *It helps you predict how much glucose will be entering your bloodstream after you eat.*
- Is carb counting the same as a low-carb diet? *No. Healthy carbohydrate sources like fruits, vegetables, whole grains, and low-fat dairy foods are an important part of your daily calorie intake. Many low-carb diets restrict carbohydrate intake lower than the American Diabetes Association recommends.*

Basic Carb Counting — ②

In this chapter, you'll learn:

- How to set carb goals
- About carb choices
- How to find out how many grams of carb are in the foods you eat

How Much Carbohydrate Should I Eat?

This is a common question asked by people with diabetes. There is no one answer; there is no set amount of carbohydrate that is right for everyone. Your carb needs will be based on several factors:

- Your height and weight
- Your gender
- Your body type
- Your usual eating habits and daily schedule
- The foods you like to eat
- Your amount of physical activity
- Your health status and diabetes goals
- Your weight goals (maintaining weight or losing weight)
- If you take diabetes medications and, if so, the times that you take them
- Your blood glucose monitoring results
- The results of your blood lipid (cholesterol and triglyceride) tests

What Is a Carb Choice?

Many carb counters find that it is easier to count carb "choices" than grams. Here's how the carb choice method works: one carb choice equals 15 grams of carbohydrate. So, if your goal is 60 grams of carb per meal, that would translate to four carb choices per meal.

Here are some examples of foods and serving sizes that count as one carb choice:
- 1 cup low-fat milk
- 1 small apple
- 1 slice of bread

Table 2.1 shows more examples of common food portions that contain 15 grams of carbohydrate. Of course, in the real world, not all carb choices contain *exactly* 15 grams of carbohydrate. This amount is used as a handy "rule of thumb" for carb counting.

If you eat more than the portion size listed, you'll need to count more than one carb choice. For example, Table 2.1 shows that half a grapefruit counts as one carb choice. If you eat the whole grapefruit, that counts as two carb choices. You also may eat more than one food that counts as a carb choice in a meal. For example, based on Table 2.1, if you ate half a grapefruit and ate 3/4 cup of plain yogurt in the same meal, that would count as two carb choices for the meal.

You don't have to use carb choices to do carb counting—you can also just count the individual grams of carb in the foods you eat and keep track that way. You can decide which works best for you.

Table 2.1 Examples of Food Portions That Equal 1 Carb Choice
(15 g Carbohydrate)

Food/beverage	Serving size
White rice, cooked	1/3 cup
Pasta, cooked	1/3 cup
Grapefruit	1/2 a fruit
Yogurt, plain	3/4 cup

Rely on an Expert

You don't have to figure out this carb counting thing all on your own! If you decide you want to try carb counting, a specially trained clinician can be a valuable addition to your diabetes care team. Here are some credentials to look for:

- CDE (Certified Diabetes Educator): registered dietitians (RDs), registered nurses (RNs), physicians, and other health care professionals are eligible for this credential.
- BC-ADM (Board Certified–Advanced Diabetes Management): this credential is available to RDs, RNs, physicians, physician assistants (PAs), and registered pharmacists.

Both credentials require extensive experience and training, continuous education, and passing a certification examination.

To find CDEs and BC-ADMs in your area, ask your diabetes care provider or check out these resources:

- American Diabetes Association
  Visit www.diabetes.org/findaprogram and enter your zip code.
  Or call 1-800-DIABETES (1-800-342-2383).
- American Association of Diabetes Educators
  Visit www.diabeteseducator.org and click on Find an Education Program at the top of the page.

Diabetes education isn't just about carb counting. A specialist can help you learn more about many different aspects of diabetes and your self-management efforts. Diabetes education is so important, Medicare and many private health insurance policies now cover individual or group sessions. Check the details on your coverage—it may be referred to as *diabetes self-management education* (DSME), *diabetes self-management training* (DSMT), or *nutrition counseling for diabetes* (also referred to as medical nutrition therapy, or MNT).

Ideally, your diabetes care provider referred you to diabetes education when you were first diagnosed. If not, ask at your next appointment. Effective diabetes care depends on your self-management skills—and the best way to learn is with an experienced teacher and guide at your side.

How Do You Know How Many Grams of Carbohydrate Are in the Foods You Eat?

Fortunately, it's easier than ever to find out how many grams of carb are in the foods we eat. There are many resources available today, from smartphone apps to websites, to books and pocket guides. Appendix 2 at the back of this book lists some of them. There is also the Nutrition Facts label on packaged foods, and the nutrition information listed with many recipes and on restaurant menus and websites. In the next chapter, we'll dive into the Nutrition Facts label in detail. For now, let's just look at where you can find the carbohydrate information on labels, recipes, and restaurant websites.

Nutrition Facts Label

Every packaged food in the grocery store is required to have a Nutrition Facts label. For basic carb counting, you want to focus on two pieces of information:

- The serving size
- The grams of total carbohydrate

Figure 2.1 shows where to find both. This is a sample Nutrition Facts label for a 1/2 cup serving of regular Cream of Wheat cooked with water. As you can see, this food contains 13.8 grams of total carb in a 1/2 cup serving.

We know that 15 grams of carbohydrate equals one choice. So one serving of this food would count for one carb choice.

If you ate two servings, it would count as two carb choices:

$$\begin{array}{r} 13.8 \text{ grams of carbohydrate} \\ \times \quad 2 \text{ servings} \\ \hline = \quad 27.6 \text{ grams of carbohydrate} \end{array}$$

27.6 grams of carbohydrate/15 = 1.84 carb choices (round up to 2)

Nutrition Facts	
2 servings per container	
Serving size	**1/2 cup (126g)**
Amount per serving	
Calories	**65**
	% Daily Value*
Total Fat 0.3g	**<1%**
Saturated Fat <0.1g	**<1%**
Trans Fat 0g	
Cholesterol 0mg	**0%**
Sodium 4mg	**<1%**
Total Carbohydrate 13.8g	**5%**
Dietary Fiber 0.6g	**3%**
Total Sugars <0.1g	
Protein 1.9g	
Vitamin D 0mcg	0%
Calcium 58mg	4%
Iron 4.7mg	26%
Potassium 21mg	<1%

*The % Daily Value (DV) tells you how much a nutrient in a serving of food contributes to a daily diet. 2000 calories a day is used for general nutrition advice.

Figure 2.1 Nutrition Facts label for a serving of Cream of Wheat.

As you can see from the equations above, you may need to do some math if you eat a different amount of the food than what is listed on the label. (Many of the nutritional information apps and websites available today will do the calculations for you if you change the serving size, as shown in Fig. 2.3.)

There are many sources available to help you learn how many grams of carb are in the foods you eat.

Recipes

Many recipes on websites and in magazines include nutritional information at the bottom. As on Nutrition Facts labels, the nutrition information in the recipe should list the serving size and the grams of carb in one serving. Figure 2.2 is an example from the American Diabetes Association's website DiabetesFoodHub.org.

This recipe for Pesto Chicken Kabobs contains 9 grams of carbohydrate in one serving. One serving equals two skewers (or kabobs). So four skewers would provide 18 grams of carbohydrate, or one carb choice.

The recipe recommends serving the kabobs with a Quinoa Pilaf on the side (also a recipe from the website). But what if you want to prepare a side of plain quinoa? A package of quinoa should include a Nutrition Facts label, or you could look up the nutritional info on a website. For this example, let's look up quinoa on CalorieKing.com.

In Fig. 2.3, you can see that you can change the serving size. We changed the measurement to cup, and entered 0.33 for 1/3 cup of cooked quinoa. The website does the calculation for us and tells us that 1/3 cup of cooked quinoa contains 13 grams of carbohydrate. This total equals one carb choice. So, if you had four of the Pesto Chicken Kabobs along with 1/3 cup of cooked quinoa, altogether that would be 31 grams of carbohydrate, or two carb choices.

Restaurant Menus and Websites

Many restaurants now provide nutritional information on their printed menus, menu boards, and/or websites. Menus may only list calories, not total carbohydrate, but some places have more detailed information available in printed form if you ask, or you can find more nutritional details on their website. Some chain restaurants even have smartphone apps with nutritional information. Figure 2.4 shows nutrition information for blueberry oatmeal available on Starbucks' website, and this example shows the total carbohydrate.

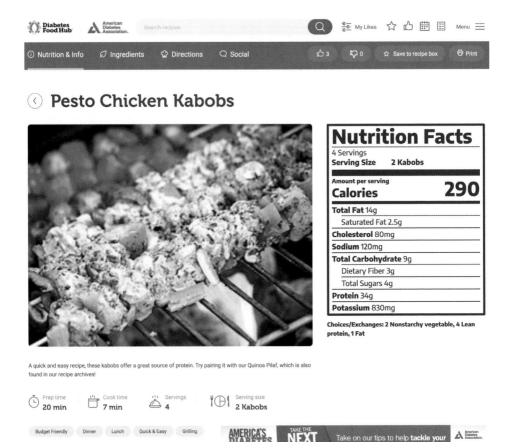

Figure 2.2 Recipe for Pesto Chicken Kabobs, taken from the American Diabetes Association website DiabetesFoodHub.org.

In Chapter 8, we'll talk more about how to use carb counting when eating at restaurants. For now, just be aware that there are many sources available to help you learn how many grams of carbohydrate are in the foods you eat.

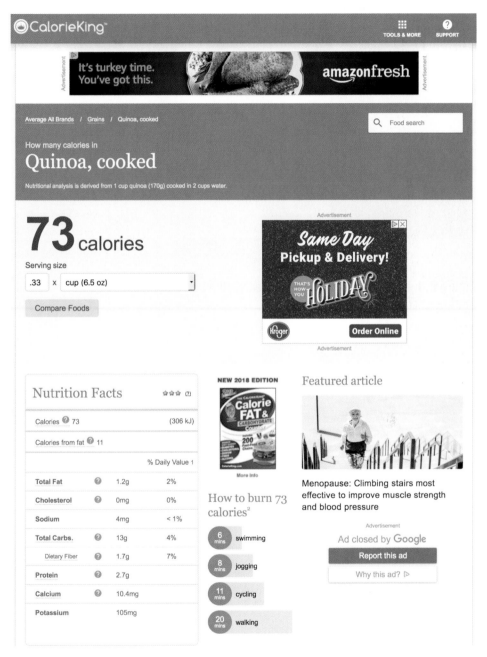

Figure 2.3 Breakdown of a recipe serving size for quinoa, taken from CalorieKing.com/foods/.

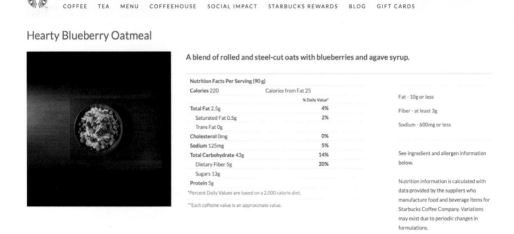

Figure 2.4 Nutrition information for Hearty Blueberry Oatmeal, taken from Starbucks.com, June 2018.

Let's Review

See if you can answer these questions. Refer back to the chapter if you need help.

- What is a carb choice? *15 grams of carbohydrate*
- How can you know how many grams of carb are in the foods you eat?
  By reading food labels and checking recipes and nutritional databases
- What are the two most important pieces of information on a food label?
  Serving size and total grams of carbohydrate

Let's Practice

- Go to your pantry or refrigerator and look at the Nutrition Facts labels on some of your favorite foods. Find the serving size and the grams of total carbohydrate. How many carb choices are in one serving?
- Look at a recipe in one of your favorite cookbooks, food magazines, or websites. Does it list serving size and grams of total carbohydrate? If so, how many carb choices are in one serving?
- Look at the website of one of your favorite chain restaurants. Do they have nutritional information available? Does it include grams of total carbohydrate?

The Food Label Has the Facts

In Chapter 2, we showed you where to find the total carbohydrate grams on the Nutrition Facts label. But the label has much more information to offer. In this chapter, we'll show you how to unpack all the information on the label and teach you more about how it can help you with carb counting and healthy meal planning.

What's on the Nutrition Facts Label?

The Nutrition Facts label contains a wealth of information, based on analysis conducted by the U.S. Food and Drug Administration (FDA). Food manufacturers are required to include this label on all packaged foods. Its format is updated every so often to reflect the latest research on nutrition and public health. The examples in this book reflect the Nutrition Facts label format introduced in 2016. The new design is intended to make the label easier to read and understand and to include more of the information we all need to make healthy choices. Let's look at each item on the label in more detail. Figure 3.1 shows you an example of a Nutrition Facts label.

Servings per Container

Remember, the calories and other nutrient amounts listed on the label are for **one serving**, not for the whole

Nutrition Facts

8 servings per container

Serving Size   **2/3 cup (55g)**

Amount per serving

Calories   **230**

	% Daily Value*
Total Fat 8g	**10%**
Saturated Fat 1g	**5%**
Trans Fat 0g	
Cholesterol 0mg	**0%**
Sodium 160mg	**7%**
Total Carbohydrate 37g	**13%**
Dietary Fiber 4g	**14%**
Total Sugars 12g	
Includes 10g Added Sugars	**20%**
Protein 3g	
Vitamin D 2mcg	10%
Calcium 260mg	20%
Iron 8mg	45%
Potassium 235mg	6%

*The % Daily Value (DV) tells you how much a nutrient in a serving of food contributes to a daily diet. 2000 calories a day is used for general nutrition advice.

Figure 3.1 Sample Nutrition Facts label.

container (unless the container is single-serve). Not taking into account the multiple servings is an easy mistake to make when you first start reading food labels. If there is more than one serving per container, you'll need to multiply all of the other nutritional information by the number of servings you eat.

Serving Size

Serving sizes for categories of food are set by the FDA, so serving sizes are consistent among different manufacturers. Serving sizes are also listed both in common household amounts (such as 4 crackers or 3/4 cup of pasta) as well as metric measures (for example, 28 grams).

Calories

This is the number of calories in **one serving**, listed in large, bold print.

% Daily Value

Daily values are average levels of nutrients recommended for a person eating 2,000 calories a day. For example, the recommended daily value of calcium is 1,000 mg for adults and children 4 years of age and older. The % Daily Value column on the Nutrition Facts label tells you how much one serving of that food contributes to the recommended daily value of that nutrient. For example, a food with 200 mg calcium in a serving would contribute 20% toward the daily value of 1,000 mg. Remember, these are just average guidelines. Your diabetes care team may recommend different nutrient levels for you based on a variety of factors.

Total Fat

The Total Fat listing includes the grams of Saturated Fat and Trans Fat, explained on the following page.

Saturated Fat

The grams of saturated fat are indented under Total Fat because they are included in the Total Fat number. In this example, the label tells us that one serving of this food has 8 grams of fat, and 1 of those 8 grams is saturated fat. In general, it is best to limit saturated fat because of its connection with heart disease and other health problems.

Trans Fat

Because U.S. food manufacturers are no longer permitted to use trans fats in their products, you shouldn't see this item on food labels much longer. Trans fats are man-made fats that have been widely used in food manufacturing for decades. However, in the 1990s, research began to suggest a significant link between trans fats and heart disease. The final trans fat ban went into effect in June 2018. If you see a food label with trans fats listed, know this: it is best to avoid foods that contain this ingredient.

Cholesterol

Cholesterol indicates the milligrams of cholesterol in one serving.

Sodium

Sodium indicates the milligrams of sodium in one serving.

Total Carbohydrate

All of the grams of carbohydrate in one serving are listed. *This is the number that you should look at when you count carbohydrate.* The Total Carbohydrate listing includes the grams of Dietary Fiber and Total Sugars, explained below.

Dietary Fiber

The grams of dietary fiber per serving are indented under Total Carbohydrate, because these grams are included in the Total Carbohydrate number. In this example, one serving of this food contains 37 grams of carbohydrate, and 4 of those grams are made up of dietary fiber.

Total Sugars

The grams of sugars per serving are also indented under Total Carbohydrate because these grams are included in the Total Carbohydrate number. Remember, there are many kinds of sugars: lactose, glucose, and fructose, just to name a few. Total sugars includes the grams of all kinds of sugars, whether they occur naturally in foods (like lactose in dairy products) or are added during preparation (like high fructose corn syrup). Sometimes people with diabetes focus on the grams of total sugar on the food label, rather than the grams of total carbohydrate. But remember, all types of carbohydrate are broken down into glucose, and your body can't tell the difference. For carb counting, the item you want to focus on is Total Carbohydrate. For more information about the different kinds of sugar and sweeteners, see Nutritional Claims on page 23.

Added sugars

Under Total Sugars, this example says "Includes 10g Added Sugars." This listing was added to the Nutrition Facts label in the 2016 revision to help people better understand the amounts and sources of sugars in their foods. Added sugars are things like white sugar and brown sugar (sucrose) and high fructose corn syrup that are added to prepared foods during processing. This label tells us that out of the 12 grams of Total Sugars in one serving of this food, 10 of those grams are from sugars added to the food during processing.

Protein

Protein indicates the grams of protein in one serving.

Vitamins and Minerals

Under the third bold line, the Nutrition Facts label lists a variety of vitamins and minerals. The FDA requires that food labels include listings for vitamin D, calcium, iron, and potassium. If the food manufacturer makes any claims about other vitamins or minerals in its packaging, it must include that nutrient on its Nutrition Facts label as well. For example, if a cereal's package says it is a "good source of folic acid," folic acid must be included on its label. (For more information, see the Nutritional Claims section.) As you see in Fig. 3.1, some nutrients will be listed in micrograms (mcg) and some in milligrams (mg). The percentages listed next to them in the right-hand column are the % Daily Value, which tells you how much one serving of that food contributes to the recommended daily value of that nutrient. (For more information, see % Daily Value above.)

The Nutrition Facts label contains a lot of information. But remember, for basic carb counting, you only need to focus on the serving size and the grams of Total Carbohydrate. That's it! Those two pieces of information can get you well on your way to managing your blood glucose, feeling your best, and preventing diabetes complications.

Diabetes experts agree that total carbohydrate is the most important information for carb counters.

Nutritional Claims

Food manufacturers know that many people are trying to eat more healthfully, for a variety of reasons. As a result, we're seeing more and more nutritional claims in food advertising and on food packaging. These are words printed on the food package, separate from the Nutrition Facts label. If you start looking, you'll find a lot of examples: "fat free," "sugar free," "a good source of fiber," etc.

Let's look at a few common areas of nutritional claims that come into play with carb counting.

Fiber

Remember, dietary fiber is a type of carbohydrate. On the Nutrition Facts label, it is listed under Total Carbohydrate. When using carb counting, you won't count grams of dietary fiber separately. But fiber is an important nutrient for overall good health, and research shows that many people don't get enough fiber in their diets. The FDA regulates what manufacturers can say about their foods based on how many grams of dietary fiber are provided per serving. Table 3.1 lists the required number of grams for each phrase.

Whole Grains

You've probably heard or read about the nutritional value of whole grains. Whole grains have been associated with better heart health and lower cancer risk, among other benefits.

All grains are made up of three parts: the bran, the germ, and the endosperm. The endosperm is the part that contains starch. Products are called "whole grain" when they are made from flour that contains all three parts of the grain. The opposite

Table 3.1 Fiber Claims on the Food Label

Fiber claim	Means
High or excellent source per serving	≥5 g fiber
Good source	2.5–4.9 g per serving
More, enriched, or added	At least 2.5 g per serving

Source: *Guidance for Industry: A Food Labeling Guide.* U.S. Department of Health and Human Services, Food and Drug Administration, and Center for Food Safety and Applied Nutrition, 2013.

When shopping, look for a whole grain as the first ingredient; it may say "whole wheat" or the word "whole" with another type of grain, like oats. Don't be fooled by the term "multi-grain" or "seven-grain." These phrases just mean the food contains more than one kind of grain, not that any of them are whole grains.

of this is called "refined flour": flour made mainly from the endosperm of the grain, with the bran and germ removed.

The bran and germ contain many nutrients that are good for our health. That's why health authorities, including the American Diabetes Association, recommend breads, pastas, crackers, and other baked goods made with whole-grain flour. All adults are encouraged to have three to five servings of whole grains each day; one serving is 16 grams of whole grain.

When shopping, look for a whole grain as the first ingredient; it may say "whole wheat" or the word "whole" with another type of grain, like oats. Don't be fooled by the term "multi-grain" or "seven-grain." These phrases just mean the food contains more than one kind of grain, not that any of them are whole grains. You can also look for the Whole Grain Stamp (Fig. 3.2).

As you can see in Fig. 3.2, there are three different varieties of the Whole Grain Stamp: the 100% Stamp, the 50%+ Stamp, and the Basic Stamp.

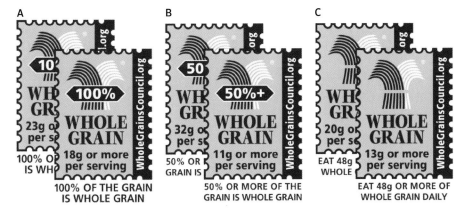

Figure 3.2 Whole-Grain Stamps. *A:* 100% Stamp. *B:* 50%+ Stamp. *C:* Basic Stamp. Reprinted with permission from the Oldways Whole Grains Council, www.WholeGrainsCouncil.org.

- The **100% Stamp** (Fig. 3.2*A*) means that all of the grain ingredients in the food are whole grain.
- The **50%+ Stamp** (Fig. 3.2*B*) means that at least half of the grain ingredients in the food are whole grain.
- The **Basic Stamp** (Fig. 3.2*C*) means that the food contains at least 8 grams (a half serving) of whole grain, but may also contain some refined grain.

Net Carb and Impact Carb

You may have heard or read about the terms "net carbs" or "impact carbs." These phrases are often used in reference to low-carb diets, which are popular for weight loss and weight management. You may see these terms used on some food packaging or in food advertisements.

To arrive at "net carbs," the manufacturers subtract the total grams of sugar alcohols and fiber from the grams of total carbohydrate in the product (you will learn more about sugar alcohols later in this chapter). The remaining grams of carbohydrate are then referred to as "net carbs." Some manufacturers also include a statement saying only the net carbs in the product have an impact on blood glucose. However, this information is often inconsistent from product to product, because this aspect of food labeling is not regulated by the FDA or any other authority.

It is also important to know that these terms and phrases are not approved or regulated by the FDA. Also, the American Diabetes Association does not use these terms. Diabetes experts agree that total carbohydrate is the most important information for carb counters.

What Is the Glycemic Index?

The glycemic index, or GI, measures how a carbohydrate-containing food raises blood glucose. In the index, foods are ranked based on how they compare to a reference food—either pure glucose, like in a glucose tablet, or white bread. A food with a high GI raises blood glucose more than a food with a medium or low GI.

Knowing the GI of a food is valuable information, but it can be difficult for people with diabetes to use the GI for blood glucose management. GI only evaluates one food at a time, and most people eat several foods in a meal. Some are high in carbohydrate and others are high in protein or fat. The combination of foods in a meal is what determines the effect on blood glucose. In addition, a number of other factors affect how quickly foods raise your blood glucose. The factors include:

- If you take blood glucose–lowering medication
- The fiber content of the foods you eat
- The ripeness of the fruit or vegetables you eat
- Whether the food is cooked or raw
- How quickly or slowly you eat
- The level of blood glucose before a meal (when the starting point is low, blood glucose rises faster after a meal)
- The time of your last dose of diabetes medication and the time you eat

For most people, carb counting is easier to use in everyday life than the glycemic index. However, some people learn to use the GI to fine-tune blood glucose management efforts over time. After gaining experience with carb counting, you may learn how certain foods affect your blood glucose more than others—your own personal GI. For now, we'll stick with carb counting basics.

Sugars

When people are first diagnosed with diabetes, they often think they won't be able to eat sweets anymore. In this situation, some people seek out the "sugar-free" or "no-sugar-added" foods in the supermarket. But as you're learning, it's also possible

Table 3.2 Sugar-Related Nutritional Claims

Nutrition claim	Meaning
Sugar-free	Less than 0.5 g sugars per serving
Reduced sugars	At least 25% less sugar than the regular food
No added sugar, without added sugar, no high fructose corn syrup	These claims are allowed if no amount of sugars or ingredient that substitutes for sugar is used, contains no fruit juice concentrate or jelly, and the label says the food is not low calorie

Source: *Guidance for Industry: A Food Labeling Guide.* U.S. Department of Health and Human Services, Food and Drug Administration, and Center for Food Safety and Applied Nutrition, 2013.

to fit foods sweetened with regular sweeteners into your diabetes eating plan, as long as it is in moderation. The choice is up to you.

There are lots of sugar-related claims in food advertisements and packaging. "Sugar-free," "no sugar added," and "no high fructose corn syrup" are a few examples you may have seen. Table 3.2 shows some of the nutrition claims related to sugar that are regulated by the FDA.

The whole issue of sugars in foods and drinks can be confusing because there are so many different kinds of sweeteners used in food manufacturing. Some have carbohydrate and calories and some do not. Carb counters need to know which sweeteners contain carbs and how to count them. Let's look at the different kinds of sweeteners used in foods and drinks.

> *It's also possible to fit foods sweetened with regular sweeteners into your diabetes eating plan, as long as it is in moderation. The choice is up to you.*

Nutritive sweeteners

Nutritive sweeteners contain calories and carbohydrate. In fact, all of them contain the same amount: 4 calories per gram and 4 grams of carbohydrate per level teaspoon. Table 3.3 lists common types of nutritive sweeteners in food. There are others you may read about, such as maltose, corn sugar, and high fructose corn syrup. Many of them end in "-ose." *The important thing to remember is that they all*

Table 3.3 Nutritive Sweeteners

Food	Type of sugar	Calories per gram	Grams of carb per teaspoon
Table sugar, brown sugar, powdered sugar	Sucrose	4	4
Whole fruit	Fructose	4	4
Honey	Fructose and dextrose	4	4
Molasses	Sucrose, fructose, and dextrose	4	4
Milk and other dairy	Lactose	4	4

have the same amount of calories and carbohydrate, and all are broken down into glucose in the bloodstream in the same way. All kinds of nutritive sweeteners are included in the Total Sugars figure on the Nutrition Facts label, which is part of the Total Carbohydrate listing.

Nonnutritive sweeteners (sugar substitutes)

Nonnutritive sweeteners are compounds that add sweetness to foods and drinks without adding calories or carbohydrate. You may also hear them called sugar substitutes, artificial sweeteners, or low-calorie sweeteners—they're all the same thing. Table 3.4 shows eight sugar substitutes currently approved by the FDA with their scientific names and brand names.

Sugar substitutes are used in many foods and beverages today, including diet sodas, fruit drinks, "sports" drinks, syrups, and yogurts. These sweeteners can greatly lower the carbohydrate and calories in foods. They do not, on their own, cause a rise in blood glucose levels. But be aware—foods sweetened with sugar substitutes may or may not contain carbohydrate and calories from other ingredients. For example, a yogurt may be sweetened with sucralose but may also contain carbohydrate from the fruit in it. Also, some brands may combine a sugar substitute with a sugar alcohol; see the section on page 29 for more information on sugar alcohols and their impact on blood glucose.

Nonnutritive sweeteners or sugar substitutes are not included on the Nutrition Facts label. However, you can see them listed by name in the ingredients list, and many products include the sugar substitute's name on their packaging.

Table 3.4 FDA-Approved Nonnutritive Sweeteners and Sugar Substitutes

Scientific name	Brand names
Acesulfame-potassium (or acesulfame-K)	Sunett, Sweet One, Sweet & Safe
Advantame	N/A
Aspartame	NutraSweet, Equal, Spoonful, Equal-Measure, Canderel, Benevia, AminoSweet, NatraTaste
Neotame	Newtame
Saccharin	Sweet'N Low, Necta Sweet, Cologran, Heremesetas, Sucaryl, Sucron, Sugar Twin, Sweet 10
Sucralose	Splenda
Stevia (or rebiana, rebaudioside A, or Reb-A)	Truvia (also contains sugar alcohols); SweetLeaf, PureVia
Monk fruit (or Luo Han Guo)	Fruit-Sweetness, Go-Luo, Purefruit

Sugar alcohols

Sugar alcohols (or polyols) are another type of sweetener used in sugar-free foods. They contain, on average, half the calories and carbohydrate of nutritive sweeteners. Polyols are often used in foods such as candy, cookies, snack bars, and ice creams. Many sugar alcohols end in "-ol"; see Table 3.5 for common sugar alcohol names.

Sugar alcohols aren't completely digested by the body—that's why they have about half the calories of sugar. For the same reason, sugar alcohols can cause a lower rise in blood glucose than regular sugars. (In some people, sugar alcohols may cause gas, cramps, and/or diarrhea. Foods with certain amounts of polyols are required by the FDA to have a label about this possible "laxative effect.")

Sugar alcohols are not always listed on the Nutrition Facts label. Some food manufacturers voluntarily include a line for sugar alcohols under Total Carbohydrate, along with Dietary Fiber and Total Sugars. If the packaging includes some sort of health claim about the presence of sugar alcohols, then they must be included in the Nutrition Facts. If you are not sure, look for the names of common sugar alcohols in the ingredients list.

Table 3.5 Sugar Alcohols

Sugar alcohol name	Calories per gram
Erythritol	0.2
Hydrogenated Starch Hydrolysates (HSH)	3.0
Isomalt	2.0
Lactitol	2.0
Maltitol	2.1
Mannitol	1.6
Sorbitol	2.6
Xylitol	2.4

A Note about Sweeteners

Some foods may contain more than one type of sweetener. Read ingredient lists carefully to find out what sweeteners are used; by law, they must all be listed. For example, the sweetener Truvia contains rebiana, a nonnutritive sweetener, and erythritol, which is a sugar alcohol.

Are Sugar Substitutes Safe?

You may have heard or read negative things about sugar substitutes. However, all of the sugar substitutes discussed in this chapter have gone through years of research and testing to be approved by the FDA. The FDA has declared all of these sugar substitutes "generally recognized as safe" (GRAS), which means that experts have agreed that they are safe for use by the public in appropriate amounts. However, the decision to use or not to use sugar substitutes is entirely up to you. If you are concerned or feel that sugar substitutes affect you negatively, you are welcome to eliminate or limit them in your eating plan.

*How to Include Sugar Alcohols
in Carb Counting*

If you're using carb counting to calculate your insulin dose (discussed at length in Chapter 11) and you choose to eat foods that contain sugar alcohols, you'll need to learn how to include them in your carb counts. The first step is to identify these foods. Remember, sugar alcohols are not always listed on the Nutrition Facts label. Sometimes they are listed underneath the Total Carbohydrate line, as shown in Fig. 3.3.

If sugar alcohols are not listed under Total Carbohydrate, check the ingredients list for one or more of the names listed in Table 3.5. Ingredients are listed in order by volume, so the earlier the sugar alcohol appears in the ingredients list, the more of it there is in the food.

To include sugar alcohols in your carb count, follow the steps below.

- Locate the total carbohydrate in one serving. In this example, the total carbohydrate is 29 grams.

Nutrition Facts	
1 serving per container	
Serving size	**1 bar (60g)**
Amount per serving	
Calories	**232**
	% Daily Value*
Total Fat 12g	**20%**
Saturated Fat 7g	**60%**
Trans Fat 0g	
Cholesterol 13mg	**4%**
Sodium 50mg	**2%**
Total Carbohydrate 29g	**8%**
Dietary Fiber 0g	**0%**
Total Sugars 0g	
Sugar Alcohol 18g	
Protein 2g	
Vitamin D 0mcg	0%
Calcium 78mg	6%
Iron 1.4mg	8%
Potassium 0mg	0%

*The % Daily Value (DV) tells you how much a nutrient in a serving of food contributes to a daily diet. 2000 calories a day is used for general nutrition advice.

Figure 3.3 Sugar Alcohol grams can be found under Total Carbohydrates on a Nutrition Facts label.

- Locate the amount of sugar alcohol in one serving. In this example, the sugar alcohol is 18 grams.
- Divide the grams of sugar alcohol in half. In this example, 18 grams ÷ 2 = 9 grams.
- Subtract that amount (9 grams) from the total carbohydrate number (29). That leaves with you 20 grams of carb.
- Count 20 grams of carb for this food.

That's it! Over time, you'll become familiar with certain foods you eat that contain sugar alcohols, and take note of these calculations so you can refer to them again and again.

Let's Review

See if you can answer these questions. Refer back to the chapter if you need help.

- Is the calorie count on the Nutrition Facts label for the whole package, or for one serving? *One serving*
- Do sugar substitutes like NutraSweet and Splenda have carbohydrate in them? *No*
- How can you find out if a food contains sugar alcohols? *Look for Sugar Alcohols under Total Carbohydrate on the Nutrition Facts label, and check the ingredients list for sugar alcohols by name (listed in Table 3.5)*

Let's Practice

Work through the following examples to practice your carb counting skills.

Example 1

Figure out the grams of carbohydrate and number of carb choices in this breakfast meal:

- 2/3 cup oat bran cereal
- 1/2 cup 2% milk
- 1 Tbsp raisins

Nutrition Facts label information

Food	Serving size	Total carb (g)
Oat bran cereal	1/3 cup	19
2% Milk	1 cup	13
Raisins	1/4 cup	31

How many grams of carbohydrate are in this breakfast meal? How many carb choices? (*Answers: 53 grams carb; four carb choices*)

Example 2

Figure out how many grams of carbohydrate and how many carb choices are in this dinner meal.

- 1 box prepared frozen manicotti
- 1 cup tossed green salad
- 2 Tbsp fat-free Catalina salad dressing
- 1 small dinner roll (1 ounce)
- 1 1/4 cups sliced strawberries
- 1/2 cup frozen yogurt

Nutrition Facts label information

Food	Serving size	Total carb (g)
Frozen manicotti	1 box	41
Salad greens	1 cup	7
Fat-free Catalina dressing	2 tablespoons	11
Dinner roll	1 small roll (1 ounce)	19
Strawberries	1 1/4 cups, slices	15
Frozen yogurt	1/2 cup	26

How many grams of carbohydrate are in this dinner? How many carb choices? (*Answers: 119 grams carb; eight carb choices*)

4

Measuring Foods: A Key to Your Success

In this chapter, you'll learn:

- How to measure food and drink servings
- How much carbohydrate is in common portions of food
- How to estimate the amount of carbohydrate in portions of food you eat or drink

A healthy eating plan is built on two foundations: healthful foods and healthful portion sizes. It is possible to eat only nutritious foods and still struggle with blood glucose management and body weight. The bottom line is, it's not just a matter of *what* you eat, it's also a matter of *how much*.

It's easy to let portion sizes creep up, especially when you're just getting started with carb counting. The extra carbohydrate adds up quickly. For example, if you eat a large apple at lunch, but count the amount of carbs in a medium apple, you're consuming about 10 extra grams of carb. The same goes for proteins and fats, which add extra calories that can also add up quickly. It may seem like these extras are too small to make a difference. But extra grams of carb and extra calories on a regular basis can get in the way of reaching your goals.

In this chapter, you'll learn how to take accurate measurements of your servings and how to estimate portion sizes when your measuring tools aren't available. Remember that there is no one recommendation for the amount of carb or calories you should eat each day. You and your diabetes care team will work together to figure out what is best for you.

How to Measure Servings

If you cook and bake regularly, you're already familiar with common measurements and measurement tools. If you don't, Table 4.1 can help you get comfortable with common weights and measures.

You probably have many of the following tools in your home already. If you don't, you'll want to get them; they will be invaluable to you on your carb counting journey.

Measuring Spoons

Use a set of real measuring spoons, rather than regular silverware. Table silverware varies in size based on style and won't give you exact measurements. Measuring spoon sets usually include a 1/2 teaspoon, 1 teaspoon, 1/2 tablespoon, and 1 tablespoon.

Measuring Cups—Liquids

Use a clear glass or plastic 1- or 2-cup measuring cup so you can see through it. It should have lines showing 1/4-, 1/3-, 1/2-, 2/3-, and 3/4-cup measurements. To measure liquids correctly, set the cup down on a flat surface and look at the markings at eye level to make sure the liquid reaches the proper line.

Measuring Cups—Solids

Most sets include 1/4-, 1/3-, 1/2-, and 1-cup measuring cups. When using a measuring cup, fill it to the top and level the contents with the flat edge of a knife to remove the excess.

Table 4.1 Common Household Measurements

3 teaspoons (tsp)	=	1 tablespoon (Tbsp)		
4 Tbsp	=	1/4 cup	=	2 fl oz
8 Tbsp	=	1/2 cup	=	4 fl oz
16 Tbsp	=	1 cup	=	8 fl oz
1 cup	=	1/2 pint	=	8 fl oz
2 cups	=	1 pint	=	16 fl oz
1 oz	=	30 g (dry)		

Food Scale

A food scale is helpful for foods that are measured in ounces, such as fresh fruit, breads, baked goods, meats, fish, and cheese. There are many different kinds of food scales on the market at many different prices. A simple one that measures ounces, pounds, grams, and kilograms will work for carb counting and can cost as little as $10. (There are also fancier models that cost as much as $50, but the more affordable ones will do just fine.)

Specialized Items

If you are just getting started with carb counting or are having a difficult time controlling your portions, there are specialized tools that may help you. For example, you might want to try plates divided into separate sections or bowls with measurement markings on them. There are even food dispensers that release a set amount of food, like cereal, with a twist of a dial. New portion management

A healthy eating plan is built on two foundations: healthful foods and healthful portion sizes.

products are being released all the time. Search www.shopdiabetes.org or search for food measurement tools online, and you'll find plenty to choose from.

When to Measure

When you're just getting started with carb counting, it is helpful to measure your foods and drinks as often as possible. Don't worry; you do not have to weigh and measure foods every day forever! The more you practice measuring foods and beverages, the easier it will be to estimate correct serving sizes when you don't have these tools available.

In Chapter 5, you'll learn how to keep a food log to see the types of food you usually eat and when you eat them. While you're doing your first food logs, you can also practice measuring. Most people are surprised by how much their usual portions differ from recommended serving sizes. In today's world, it's easy to lose sight of portion size—we're surrounded by super-sized portions at restaurants and in convenience foods. That's why practicing portion measurement is so important: you need to retrain your eyes and brain to recognize a recommended portion. (We'll talk more about carb counting convenience foods in Chapter 7 and restaurant meals in Chapter 8.)

Even after you gain experience and are able to estimate portion sizes, it's a good idea to recheck every so often. You may find that over time, your estimates have grown. This step can be especially helpful if you find that your weight or your blood glucose level is going up. Also, if you add a new food, try to measure it for several weeks until you get comfortable with the portion size.

Estimating Portion Sizes

Of course, you won't always be able to measure your portions at every meal. As you get more comfortable with carb counting, you'll be able to eyeball most things. Many people find it helpful to have a mental picture to help them estimate serving sizes. The box below lists some helpful guidelines that are easy to remember.

Tips and Tricks for Estimating Portion Sizes

Thumb tip (from first knuckle)* = 1 tsp
Example: 1 tsp mayonnaise or margarine
Thumb (whole, to second knuckle) = 1 Tbsp
Example: 1 Tbsp salad dressing or cream cheese
Two fingers lengthwise = 1 ounce
Example: 1 ounce cheese or meat
Palm of hand = 3 ounces
Example: 3 ounces boneless cooked meat or fish
(a regular size deck of cards or a bar of soap are also good examples)
Woman's fist = 1 cup
Man's fist = 1 1/2 cup
Example: 1 cup of cooked rice or pasta

Of course, hand and finger sizes vary from person to person; these are based on averages.

When you're eating at home, try to use the same size plates, glasses, and bowls consistently. This step will help you judge correct portions, and you won't have to use the measuring tools so often. Try this to practice: measure a serving in a measuring cup first and then take note of how much space it takes up on a plate or in a bowl or glass. For example, try this with 1 cup of pasta, 1/2 cup of cooked oatmeal, or 1/2 cup of milk. Keep these images in your mind for next time, or take pictures with your smartphone and save them for reference. Then every so often, verify that your servings are still on target.

If these portion sizes look small on your plate or in your bowl, consider using smaller plates and bowls. As portion sizes in the U.S. have grown, so have dish and bowl sizes. The American Diabetes Association recommends 9-inch plates. This visual trick can make a big difference in making you feel satisfied and full.

You'll also want to think about how you serve food at meals. Serving food "family style"—placing full serving bowls on the table—can easily lead to extra servings. If you measure out your portion of each food in the meal before sitting down at the table, you're much more likely to stay on track.

Weighing and Measuring in the Grocery Store

Successful carb counting starts in the grocery store, where you decide what kinds of foods—and how much of those foods—will come into your kitchen. As you begin to think about reading food labels and measuring your portions, you'll also want to take note of the wealth of information available to you in the grocery store as you shop. Here are some ideas.

Fruits and Vegetables

Take advantage of the food scales that hang in the produce section of most grocery stores. You can use them to get an idea of the weight of individual fruits and vegetables that you eat. This is particularly helpful for fruits and vegetables that are measured by whole food, like bananas and baked potatoes, rather than in cups, like grapes or lettuce.

For example, in Chapter 2 you learned that a small apple has about 15 grams of carbohydrate, meaning that it counts as one carb choice. But what does "small" mean? In Appendix 1, you can see that a small apple is defined as 4 ounces. While you are learning, you can use the food scale in the grocery store to help you select small apples and get familiar with what a 4-ounce apple looks like.

The same goes for vegetables: a 3-ounce baking potato has about 18 grams of carbohydrate, a little more than one carb choice. The produce scale in the grocery store can help you select potatoes that will fit into your eating plan. Remember, those extra ounces count, even with healthful foods like fruits and vegetables. For instance, if you eat an 8-ounce apple (and some apples are that large!), you'll need to count it as two carb choices. Of course, grocery store scales are not 100% accurate—if you have a food scale in your kitchen, double-check the weights when you get home.

Meats and Cheeses

While proteins like meats and cheeses don't contain carbohydrate, you still need to manage your portions of these foods. As we talked about before, proteins contain calories and also contribute fat to your diet, both things you want to watch to maintain good health. These foods can also affect the way your body responds to the carb in your meal. We'll talk more about this in Chapter 6. But for now, know that selecting meats and cheeses with portion sizes in mind can help you make healthful choices and stay on track with your eating plan.

For example, if you buy cheese or cold cuts at the deli counter, think about how many meals you need to make before you place your order. Let that be your guide to how many ounces you buy. If you make a turkey and cheese sandwich for lunch with 2 ounces of turkey and 1 ounce of cheese, how many sandwiches are you going to make until the next time you shop? Buy just the amount you need.

The same goes for buying meat. Think about how many people you are feeding, what quantity you will lose in cooking (see Raw to Cooked: Rules of Thumb below), and how much you want for leftovers. Then use this information to estimate the amount of raw meat you need to buy. Another benefit of this approach is that you will waste less food and save money!

Raw to Cooked: Rules of Thumb

Raw meat with no bone: 4 ounces raw to get 3 ounces cooked.

Raw meat with bone: 5 ounces raw to get 3 ounces cooked.

Raw poultry with skin: 4 1/4 to 4 1/2 ounces to get 3 ounces cooked. The extra 1/4 to 1/2 ounce accounts for the skin. (Remove the skin before or after cooking.)

Here is an example for a whole chicken: Each family member needs about 3 ounces cooked chicken. There are five family members. The chicken has bones and skin, so you need to estimate that you'll need about 5 1/2 ounces of raw chicken per person. So, 5 × 5 1/2 = about 28 ounces or about 1 3/4 pounds. If you want enough for two meals, you need about 3 1/2 pounds. Do not forget a few ounces for the organs stuffed in the cavity. So, you need about a 4-pound raw chicken to feed a family of five.

Let's Review

See if you can answer these questions. Refer back to the chapter if you need help.

- Why is it important to measure your portions? *Because carb count varies based on volume*
- What kinds of tools can you use to measure your foods? *Measuring cups and spoons, food scale*
- What kinds of tools can you use to estimate portions when you can't measure? *Estimation techniques based on visuals, averaging data for similar food items*

Let's Practice

Use your new skills to work through the following examples:

- Bananas are one of your favorite breakfast foods. The smartphone app you use for carb counting only has one entry for bananas, at 4 ounces. How can you figure out how to accurately count your daily banana in your carb totals?
- You're invited to a friend's wedding. The reception includes a sit-down dinner of salmon, rice, and vegetables. How can you estimate your portion sizes so you can record your carb intake when you get home?

5

Keeping Track

In this chapter, you'll learn:

- How to keep a food log
- How to identify your preferred foods and eating schedule
- How to create a food database

Let's face it—life is unpredictable. Work, travel, family, friends, volunteer commitments—many people's schedules are packed with all this and more. How can you manage your blood glucose with carb counting in the middle of all that busy-ness?

In this chapter, we'll teach you a step-by-step process to work carb counting into your real life. You'll learn how to develop an eating plan that fits your schedule, preferences, and habits and that's flexible enough for last-minute surprises. It's easier than you think!

What Are Your Current Eating Habits?

Before you set off on a new path, you need to know where you're starting from. Carb counting will be easier and more successful if you start with an honest, accurate assessment of your current eating habits and schedule. This step will help you and your diabetes care team come up with a realistic eating plan that you'll be more likely to stick with over the long term. It will also help you learn more about how what you eat and when you eat it affects your blood glucose levels and the way that you feel. Here's how to do it.

Step 1: Record Everything You Eat and Drink for 1 Week

The first step is to keep a food diary or log for 7 days. Record everything you eat and drink throughout the day, including snacks (even just a nibble). Be honest—this is not about judging your food choices. It is about gathering information to help you and your care team manage your blood glucose levels.

There are many different formats and tools you can use to keep a food log. Some people prefer writing it down with pen and paper. Others like to use a smart-phone app or website. Appendix 2 at the back of this book includes a list of apps and website tools that can help. It doesn't matter what tool you use, as long as you keep up with it and include the following information:

- Day of the week
- Meal time
- Type of food or drink
- Amounts of food or drink

Let's look at a 1-day example in Table 5.1. Notice that the amounts listed are pretty specific—cups, tablespoons, ounces. The more precise you can be, the more helpful your food records will be to you and to your diabetes care provider. Remember all the measuring skills you learned in Chapter 4 and put them to good use!

Carb counting will be easier and more successful if you start with an honest, accurate assessment of your current eating habits and schedule.

Step 2: Find the Foods You Ate That Contain Carbohydrate

After you have 1 week of your food diary completed, go through each day and circle or highlight the foods that contain at least 1 gram of carbohydrate. You can identify these foods by using Appendix 1 or by using one or more of the resources listed in Appendix 2. See Table 5.2 for an example. As you can see, it's not just the rice, bread, and desserts that contain carbs; dairy foods and fruits contain carbs, and even salad dressing may contain a few grams. The only

Table 5.1 Sample Food Diary

Day	Time	Food	Amount
Monday	7:00 a.m.	Blueberry bagel	1 medium (3.7 oz)
		Light cream cheese	2 Tbsp
		Strawberries	1 cup, sliced
	12:00 noon	Thin-crust cheese pizza (14")	3 slices
		Garden salad	1 1/2 cups
		Thousand Island dressing	2 Tbsp
		Frozen yogurt, low-fat	1/2 cup
		Sugar cone	1
	6:30 p.m.	Grilled chicken breast	5 oz, cooked
		Barbecue sauce	2 Tbsp
		Long-grain brown rice	1 cup
		Corn on the cob	1 large piece
		Margarine	2 Tbsp
		Applesauce (no sugar added)	1 cup
	9:00 p.m.	Oatmeal raisin cookie	1 large (2 oz)

foods on the diary that do not contain *some* carbohydrate are the chicken breast (a protein) and margarine (a fat).

Step 3: Figure How Much Carb You Eat

Now, go back and figure out the number of grams of carbohydrate in each of the foods you ate. Then add up the totals for each meal and snack. If you plan to use carb choices rather than grams of carbohydrate, remember that each carb choice contains about 15 grams of carbohydrate. (We show both grams and choices in Table 5.3.) Then total up how many grams of carb or carb choices you ate at each meal and over the course of each day.

Step 4: Identify Your Habits and Preferences

Once you've gone through steps 1–3 for all 7 days, you can review the whole week's logs for patterns. Do you tend to eat more carb in the morning? Do you like to have a

Table 5.2 Sample Food Diary with Carb Sources Circled

Day	Time	Food	Amount
Monday	7:00 a.m.	Blueberry bagel	1 medium (3.7 oz)
		Light cream cheese	2 Tbsp
		Strawberries	1 cup, sliced
	12:00 noon	Thin-crust cheese pizza (14")	3 slices
		Garden salad	1 1/2 cups
		Thousand Island dressing	2 Tbsp
		Frozen yogurt, low-fat	1/2 cup
		Sugar cone	1
	6:30 p.m.	Grilled chicken breast	5 oz, cooked
		Barbecue sauce	2 Tbsp
		Long-grain brown rice	1 cup
		Corn on the cob	1 large piece
		Margarine	2 Tbsp
		Applesauce (no sugar added)	1 cup
	9:00 p.m.	Oatmeal raisin cookie	1 large (2.5 oz)

snack after dinner? Do you generally eat at the same times each day, or does it vary? Taking your habits and preferences into account in your eating plan will help you feel satisfied and motivated to stick with it. Be honest with your diabetes care team about your preferences and the realities of your life.

Step 5: Create a Meal Database

Most of us are creatures of habit—we eat the same foods day in and day out. That's good news when it comes to carb counting because it makes it easier to build your own personal database or library of carb counts. You can save time in the long run by spending a few minutes developing a database of the carb counts of your common meals. For example, you may find that for breakfast, you usually eat either an egg sandwich, or a yogurt and a banana. Because you eat those meals

Table 5.3 Sample Food Diary with Grams of Carb and Carb Choices

Day	Time	Food	Amount	Grams of carb	Carb choices (15 g each)
Monday	7:00 a.m.	Blueberry bagel	1 medium (3.7 oz)	58	4
		Light cream cheese	2 Tbsp	2	N/A
		Strawberries	1 cup, sliced	13	1
Total				73 grams	5
	12:00 noon	Thin-crust cheese pizza (14")	3 slices	50	3 1/2
		Garden salad	1 1/2 cups	7	1/2
		Thousand Island dressing	2 Tbsp	5	1/2
		Frozen yogurt, low-fat	1/2 cup	23	1 1/2
		Sugar cone	1	8	1/2
Total				93	6 1/2
	6:30 pm	Grilled chicken breast	5 oz, cooked		
		Barbecue sauce	2 Tbsp	4	N/A
		Long-grain brown rice	1 cup	45	3
		Corn on the cob	1 large piece	32	2
		Margarine	2 Tbsp		
		Applesauce (no sugar added)	1 cup	28	2
Total				109	7
	9:00 p.m.	Oatmeal raisin cookie	1 large (2.5 oz)	32	2
Total				32	2
Total for the day				307	About 20 1/2

N/A, not applicable.

regularly, it will become easy to remember their total carb counts. Some meal tracking apps and websites even let you save and name meals you eat frequently (for example, Breakfast 1, Breakfast 2) to make it even easier. Many also allow you to mark certain foods as favorites, so they are easier to find quickly. If you prefer to keep your food log in a notebook or computer spreadsheet, you can do the same manually. Table 5.4 shows an example.

Table 5.4 Sample Personal Database: My Common Meals and Snacks

Meal	Serving (amount I eat)	Grams of carbohydrate*
BREAKFAST 1 (AT HOME)		
Honey-flavored O's cereal	1 cup	24
Bran cereal with extra fiber	1/2 cup	23
Milk, nonfat	1 cup	12
Blueberries	1/2 cup	10
Total		69
BREAKFAST 2 (IN THE CAR)		
Whole-wheat toast (for egg sandwich)	2 slices	26
Egg (fried in nonstick skillet)	1 large	0
Cheddar cheese, reduced-fat	1 oz	0
Banana	1 medium (4 oz)	27
Total		53
LUNCH		
Whole-wheat bread	2 slices	26
Smoked turkey, sliced	2 oz	0
Swiss cheese, part-skim	1 oz	1
Baby carrots	7–10	8
Grape tomatoes	5–8	3
Apple, Granny Smith	1 large (7 oz)	29
Total		67

*Nutrition information obtained from www.ars.usda.gov/nutrientdata (the USDA searchable database; for more information about this database, see Appendix 2) and Nutrition Facts labels.

Step 6: Figure Out Your Carb Intake Targets

Now you have a picture of how much carbohydrate you usually eat at your meals and snacks. Next you need to determine whether the amount you're eating is too much, too little, or just about right. Your target carbohydrate intake will vary based on a variety of factors. Talk to your diabetes care provider to set carb choice goals that are right for you.

Let's Review

See if you can answer these questions. Refer back to the chapter if you need help.

- What are the four pieces of information you should include in your first food logs? *Day of the week, meal time, type of food or drink, amounts of food or drink*
- What are three different tools you could use to maintain your carb counting records? *On paper, smartphone app, website*

Let's Practice

Use your new skills to work through these examples.

- Identify one breakfast meal and one lunch meal that you eat regularly. Create a food log entry for this meal. Don't forget to include drinks and condiments. Any surprises? How does its carb count compare to your targets?
- If you find that these meals are above or below the carb count targets, note ways you can modify those favorite meals to make them fit the goal. Write down those ideas so you can review them with your diabetes care provider or certified diabetes educator.

6

Protein, Fat, and Alcohol Count, Too

In this chapter, you'll learn:

- About protein and fat in your eating plan
- How protein and fat affect blood glucose
- How to incorporate alcohol into your eating plan (if desired)

So far, we've focused almost exclusively on carbohydrate. But in real life, we consume lots of other types of food and drink. What about the other types of nutrients in your food, like protein and fat? What about beer, wine, and mixed drinks?

All of these can be part of a balanced, healthy eating plan, and all of them can be accounted for in carb counting. As we said before, a healthy eating plan for a person with diabetes is just like a healthy eating plan for any adult—low in saturated fat and high in fiber, with a variety of fruits, vegetables, and lean proteins, and minimal processed foods. Carb counters just need to keep their eyes on one other thing—how these foods and drinks affect their blood glucose.

Protein and Fat

When protein and fats are eaten in recommended amounts, they have little effect on blood glucose levels. But there are some important reasons to pay attention to protein and fat in your meals:

- Protein and fat contain calories, and all calories count. Remember, this is true for everyone, not just for people with diabetes.

- Too much protein, especially animal protein, and too much fat, especially saturated fat and trans fat, are not healthy for anyone—but especially for people with diabetes. A diet high in animal protein and fat has been linked to higher rates of heart disease, and people with diabetes are already at a higher risk for heart disease.
- Meals high in fat and protein—like an 8-ounce steak or fried chicken—may cause your blood glucose to rise more slowly than usual and peak later than expected. This is especially important if you're using carb counting to help determine your insulin dose. (We'll talk more about using carb counting with medications in Chapter 10 and Chapter 11.) If you use insulin, talk with your diabetes care provider about how protein and fat may affect your dosage calculations.

The Need for Protein and Fat

Protein is made up of amino acids that the body needs to build muscle. Our bodies also need some fat to carry the fat-soluble vitamins A, D, E, and K; to cushion the body's vital organs; and to provide insulation to keep us warm. But most people consume more protein and fat than the body needs to conduct its business, and many people choose to eat less-than-healthy protein and fat sources.

Which Foods Contain Protein?

Many people would answer "red meat, poultry, and seafood," which is correct. But protein turns up in other foods, too. Many of these other sources contain a combination of protein and carbohydrate or protein and fat. For example, many beans and peas contain protein and carbohydrate. Nuts contain protein and fat. There are also a variety of soy-based proteins on the market, like tofu and tempeh. These products are usually lower in fat than meat, but also contain carbohydrate.

Which Foods Contain Fat?

Some foods are just about 100% fat, such as butter, margarine, oil, or regular salad dressing. These foods are often added to other foods to make them taste better—that's why we call them "added fats." On average, one serving of these types of foods contains about 5 grams of fat and 45 calories. Other foods, such as meats, cheese, nuts, whole-milk dairy foods, and most desserts, get some (but not all) of their calories from fat. You might call these "attached fats," where fat is naturally part of the food. In fat-containing foods, the fat is made up of varying amounts of three types of fat—saturated, polyunsaturated, and monounsaturated. Table 6.1 shows the different types of fat, their actions in the body, and their food sources. When it comes to dietary fat, it's a question of quality over quantity: choose healthy monounsaturated and polyunsaturated fats in moderation, and limit saturated fats.

People with diabetes have a two to four times greater risk of developing heart disease than people without diabetes. The best way to reduce this risk is to reduce your intake of all fats, with a special focus on saturated fats.

Table 6.1 Dietary Fats

Type of fat	Positive action	Negative action	Sources
Monounsaturated	Lowers total cholesterol		Oils (liquid canola, olive, and peanut)
Polyunsaturated			
Omega-3	Lowers risk of heart disease; lowers triglyceride levels		Fatty fish (salmon, sardines, herring, albacore tuna); ground flax and flaxseed oil; soybean oil, canola oil, walnuts
Omega-6	Lowers total cholesterol	Lowers HDL or "good" cholesterol	Oils (liquid corn, safflower, soybean)
Saturated		Raises total and LDL or "bad" cholesterol	Beef, pork, butter, whole-milk dairy

What Is the Mediterranean Diet?

You may have read or heard references to the "Mediterranean Diet" in recent years. This term is used to describe the traditional eating patterns of people who live near the Mediterranean Sea: a diet with lots of vegetables and whole grains, with protein from fish and poultry rather than red meat. Generally, the Mediterranean Diet contains 50% of daily calories from carbohydrates and about 30% of calories from fats (mostly healthy fats from olive oil; saturated fats are kept under 10% of daily calories). Research has shown that the Mediterranean Diet is a healthy eating pattern for people with type 2 diabetes.

How Much Protein Should You Eat?

For most people with diabetes, the guidelines for daily protein intake are the same as for other adults: 15–20% of your daily calories. The Recommended Daily Allowance (RDA) of protein for the average male is about 42 grams and, for the average female, it's about 35 grams. (Because each ounce of protein food contains about 7 grams of protein, those guidelines translate to about 6 ounces of protein daily for men and 5 ounces of protein daily for women.) The amount of fat and calories in that protein serving will vary, depending on the type of protein you choose (see Table 6.2).

How Much Fat Should You Eat?

This is another area where the nutrition guidance for people with diabetes is the same as for everyone else. Federal nutrition guidelines recommend getting less than 30% of total daily calories from all types of fat and limiting saturated fats specifically to less than 10% of your total daily calories. As for trans fat, all people are encouraged to eliminate them from their diets as much as possible.

Table 6.2 Fat and Calories for Meat Servings

Type of meat (3 oz, cooked)	Fat (g)	Calories
Lean meat (tenderloin, chicken, flounder)	9	165
Medium-fat meats (ground beef, pork chops)	15	225
High-fat meats (pork ribs)	24	300

A Note about Reduced-Fat and Fat-Free Products

The push to eat less fat has led to the availability of reduced-fat, low-fat, and fat-free versions of foods, such as ice cream, sour cream, cream cheese, salad dressing, potato chips, and margarine. When fat is removed from food to lower the fat content and calories, food manufacturers put "fat replacers" into the products to make them taste good. Fat replacers may be made from carbohydrate, protein, or fat, but the majority of fat replacers in use today are made of carbohydrate. So the calories and fat in the food may be lower—but the carbohydrate content usually is higher. For people with diabetes, these extra grams of carbohydrate can affect blood glucose levels.

If you want to try some of these products, read the Total Carbohydrate listing on the Nutrition Facts labels to determine their carbohydrate content. Try a few. Find ones that you enjoy and help you achieve your nutrition goals. If you don't like them, don't use them—there are plenty of other ways to lower your fat intake.

What Can You Learn from the Grams of Total Fat?

Remember from Chapter 3 that the Nutrition Facts label lists grams of total fat, with saturated fat indented below it. Let's look at how you can use that information to keep your fat intake within the recommended limits. In this example, our meal plan aims for 1,500 daily calories with less than 30% of those calories coming from fat.

Total number of calories: 1,500

Multiply calories by 30%:   1,500
$$\times \quad 0.30$$
450 calories from fat

There are 9 calories in each gram of fat. So to find the grams of total fat you should aim for, divide the calories from fat by 9:

$$450 \div 9$$
50 grams of total fat

So, in a 1,500-calorie-per-day eating plan, you want to eat less than 50 grams of fat.

What about saturated fat? The recommendations say that less than 10% of your total calories should come from saturated fat. You can figure out that number, too.

Multiply calories by 10%:

$$
\begin{array}{r}
1{,}500 \\
\times \quad 0.10 \\
\hline
150 \text{ calories from fat}
\end{array}
$$

Divide this number by 9 (9 calories per gram of fat):

$$
\begin{array}{r}
150 \\
\div \quad 9 \\
\hline
\text{about 17 grams of saturated fat}
\end{array}
$$

Why Is Limiting Saturated Fat So Important for People with Diabetes?

We know that eating too much saturated fat is not a good idea for anyone. Research has shown that eating a diet high in saturated fat increases your risk for heart disease. But this is even more important for people with diabetes to remember, because people with diabetes have a two to four times greater risk of developing heart disease than people without diabetes. Because of this statistic, your diabetes care provider will recommend that you get a blood test every year to check the cholesterol and triglyceride levels in your blood, both known markers for heart disease. The best way to reduce this risk is to reduce your intake of all fats, with a special focus on saturated fats and trans fat. If you don't know your current cholesterol and triglyceride levels, talk to your diabetes care provider.

....

Alcohol

Alcohol is not food, but it does contain calories, and some alcoholic beverages, such as beer and wine, contain carbohydrate. The calories from alcohol are more concentrated than the calories from carbohydrate: there are 7 calories per gram of alcohol versus 4 calories per gram of carbohydrate. So, the calories from alcohol can add up quickly.

Alcohol is unique in that it can both raise *and* lower blood glucose. Alcoholic drinks that contain carbohydrate on their own (like beer and wine) or mixed drinks that contain carbohydrate from syrups and juices can raise blood glucose just like a food that contains carbs. At the same time, drinking alcohol can cause a drop in blood glucose because alcohol blocks the production of glucose in the liver. (The liver contains "emergency stores" of glucose to raise your blood glucose if it drops too low.) Once the liver's stores of glucose are used up, a person who has consumed a lot of alcohol can't make more glucose right away, which can lead to dangerously low blood glucose or even death. This situation is especially dangerous if you take blood glucose–lowering medication or insulin.

Also, alcohol is processed by your liver, which is responsible for removing toxins and processing medication in your body. So if you are taking medications (for diabetes or for other conditions), drinking too much alcohol can cause damage to your liver.

We also know that too much alcohol can inhibit your judgment, making it more likely that you will stray from your eating plan, forget to check your blood glucose level, or forget to take a dose of medication.

The most important message about alcohol is to drink in moderation. General health guidelines and the American Diabetes Association recommend no more than one drink a day for women and two drinks a day for men. The definition of "one drink" can vary by type, but as a general rule, think 12 ounces of beer, 5 ounces of wine, or 1 1/2 ounces of distilled spirits like vodka or gin.

Tips for Drinking Alcohol Safely

- If you use a blood glucose meter, check your blood glucose before you drink, and more frequently than normal during the following 24 hours. It is especially important to check it before you go to sleep. Make sure your blood glucose is between 100 and 140 mg/dL before going to bed—if it is lower, eat something that contains carbohydrate and check it again.
- Set an alarm to check your blood glucose in the middle of the night. Symptoms of low blood glucose can be masked by the effects of alcohol.
- Do not drink on an empty stomach or when your blood glucose is low.
- If you drink in bars, wear an I.D. bracelet that notes you have diabetes. If you are in a setting where people are drinking alcohol, low blood glucose (hypoglycemia) may be mistaken for being drunk.
- Watch out for craft beers, which can have twice the alcohol and calories as a light beer.
- For mixed drinks, choose calorie-free drink mixers like diet soda, club soda, diet tonic water, or water.
- As with anyone with or without diabetes, do not drive after you drink alcohol.

If you choose to drink alcoholic beverages, do some research. Talk to your diabetes care provider about your drinking habits and how you can safely include an occasional drink in your eating plan.

Let's Review

See if you can answer these questions. Refer back to the chapter if you need help.

- How much protein should the average person eat each day? *15–20% of daily calories; about 42 grams (6 ounces) for men and about 35 grams (5 ounces) for women*
- How much fat should the average person eat each day? *Less than 30% of total daily calories from all types of fat; saturated fats less than 10% of total daily calories*
- Why is limiting saturated fat so important for people with diabetes? *Saturated fat increases the risk of heart disease, and people with diabetes are already at higher risk*
- Can people with diabetes drink alcoholic beverages? *Yes, but they need to count the carbs and watch how it affects their blood glucose*

Let's Practice

Use your new knowledge to work through these examples.

- If you know your daily calorie goal, figure out how much protein, total fat, and saturated fat you should be aiming for each day. If you don't know your daily calorie goal, figure it out based on a 2,000-calorie example.
- Look at the Nutrition Facts label on some of your favorite items in your pantry and refrigerator. Check out the protein and fat listings. How much saturated fat do they contain? Do they contain any trans fats?
- If you drink alcohol, look up the carb content in your favorite drink. Measure out what one recommended serving looks like and compare it to what you usually drink.

7

Carb Counting with Convenience Foods and Recipes

In this chapter, you'll learn:

- How to count carbs in convenience foods and ready-to-eat foods
- How to calculate the carb count of your favorite recipes

Some days, you need all the help you can get to put together a meal for yourself and your family. On those days, ready-to-eat and prepared foods can be a big help. Other days, you may enjoy cooking from scratch or trying a new recipe you've clipped out of a magazine.

Both of these approaches to cooking can be accommodated by carb counting. Your eating style does not have to completely change because of carb counting; in fact, when you become skilled at carb counting, you may enjoy using convenience foods or some of your old recipes even more because you'll be able to predict how the meal will affect your blood glucose level.

Convenience and Ready-to-Eat Foods

The convenience foods category includes everything from frozen pizza to a prepared entrée from the supermarket deli counter. When you count carbs, some convenience foods can actually be a blessing because they give you the carb count right on the Nutrition Facts label. However, some ready-to-eat foods don't come with a label, like supermarket deli items and fresh baked goods.

In some cases, you can get the information you need by doing a little research. But other times, you'll have to use your guesstimating skills. Let's learn how by working

Nutrition Facts

3 servings per container

Serving size   1/3 pizza (120g)

Amount per serving

Calories   320

	% Daily Value*
Total Fat 13g	**20%**
Saturated Fat 6g	**30%**
Trans Fat 0g	
Cholesterol 30mg	**10%**
Sodium 870mg	**36%**
Total Carbohydrate 35g	**12%**
Dietary Fiber 2g	**8%**
Total Sugars 7g	
Protein 14g	
Vitamin D 0mcg	0%
Calcium 270mg	20%
Iron 3.4mg	18%
Potassium 230mg	5%

*The % Daily Value (DV) tells you how much a nutrient in a serving of food contributes to a daily diet. 2000 calories a day is used for general nutrition advice.

Figure 7.1 Nutrition Facts label for a frozen cheese pizza.

through an example. Figure 7.1 shows a sample Nutrition Facts label for a frozen cheese pizza.

The label says one serving is 1/3 of the pizza. One serving has 35 grams of carbohydrate, or about two carb choices. If you eat half of the pizza, what would the carb count be?

Here's how to figure it out:

We know that 1/3 of the pizza is one serving. That means there are 3 servings in the box. One serving has 35 grams of carb. So,

35 (g of carb) × 3 (servings) = 105

total grams of carb in the whole pizza.

If you eat half the pizza, you'll have to figure 50% of the whole. So,

105 ÷ 2 = 53 grams of carb in half the pizza.

If you're using carb choices, you'll need to divide that number by 15. So,

53 ÷ 15 = 3.5 carb choices.

There you have it! If you ate half of this frozen pizza, you would count it as 53 grams of carb, or three and a half carb choices for the meal.

Let's look at another example. Figure 7.2 shows a sample Nutrition Facts label for a frozen dinner of Salisbury steak with mashed potatoes and green beans.

The label tells us that the complete dinner has 42 grams of carbohydrate or about three carb choices. For some people, that might leave room for some more carbs in the meal (remember, while carb targets for meals vary by person, most people aim for three to five carb choices per meal). You might add a salad, a cup of soup, and/or a dinner roll to get to your target.

What If There's No Food Label?

The examples above are fairly easy because you have the nutrition information right in front of you. It gets tougher when you don't have a Nutrition Facts label. Let's look at an example to see how that works.

Say you get a bagel with cream cheese on your way to work in the morning. You look at the carb count for a bagel on your carb counting app and note that a 3-ounce bagel has 46 grams of carbohydrate. You know the bagels that you buy are pretty large, but you're not sure how much they weigh.

So, how do you find nutrition information? You have a couple of choices. On your next supermarket trip, you can look for bagels that are similar in size to your go-to workday breakfast. If they are packaged, they will have a Nutrition Facts label. If they are loose, weigh one on a produce scale or ask someone at the bakery counter for a weight. Write it down, enter a note on your smartphone, or take a photo that you can refer to later.

Nutrition Facts

1 serving per container

Serving size   **1 meal (326g)**

Amount per serving

Calories   290

	% Daily Value*
Total Fat 6g	8%
Saturated Fat 2.5g	13%
Trans Fat 0g	
Cholesterol 35mg	12%
Sodium 490mg	21%
Total Carbohydrate 42g	15%
Dietary Fiber 7g	25%
Total Sugars 10g	
Includes 7g Added Sugars	14%
Protein 16g	
Vitamin D 0mcg	0%
Calcium 90mg	6%
Iron 2.6mg	15%
Potassium 1030mg	20%

*The % Daily Value (DV) tells you how much a nutrient in a serving of food contributes to a daily diet. 2000 calories a day is used for general nutrition advice.

Figure 7.2 Nutrition Facts label for a frozen dinner of Salisbury steak with mashed potatoes and green beans.

A second approach is to calculate an average from a variety of sources. Appendix 2 includes some nutritional databases you can refer to. Look up bagels on a few different sites and take an average of the amount of carbohydrate listed for the different sources. You can also check restaurant websites and add their information into your calculation. With all this information, you'll likely be very close. Then record the information in your personal database (see Chapter 5), so you'll have the information readily available next time.

Nutrition Facts

4 servings per container

Serving size   **1 bagel (99g)**

Amount per serving

Calories   **220**

     % Daily Value*

Total Fat 6g	**8%**
Saturated Fat 1g	**5%**
Trans Fat 0g	
Cholesterol 0mg	**0%**
Sodium 450mg	**20%**
Total Carbohydrate 45g	**16%**
Dietary Fiber 2g	**7%**
Total Sugars 3g	
Includes 2g Added Sugars	**4%**
Protein 3g	
Vitamin D 0mcg	0%
Calcium 40mg	4%
Iron 1mg	6%
Potassium 92mg	2%

*The % Daily Value (DV) tells you how much a nutrient in a serving of food contributes to a daily diet. 2000 calories a day is used for general nutrition advice.

Figure 7.3 Nutrition Facts label for a package of bagels.

Let's practice the averaging approach with our bagel example. Figure 7.3 is a sample Nutrition Facts label from a package of bagels. The label tells us that one of these bagels weighs about 99 grams (about 3.5 ounces). Each bagel contains 45 grams of carbohydrate or three carb choices. You eyeball it and determine that it's a bit smaller than the one you buy at the coffee shop.

Next you check out bagels on the Dunkin' Donuts website. You note that their plain bagel looks a little bigger than the bagel you buy. There is no weight listed, but it says the bagel contains 69 grams of carbohydrate, or four and a half carb choices. Since you think the size of your regular morning bagel is somewhere in between the two examples, you can take an average:

$$45 + 69 = 114 / 2 = 57$$

So you can estimate that the bagel you buy has 57 grams of carb, or almost four carb choices (3.8).

Try this again, this time with some items you might pick up at the deli counter. Maybe you regularly buy prepared coleslaw (the light vinegar-based type) and baked beans for quick weeknight side dishes. Now you're wondering about their carb counts, but they don't come with a Nutrition Facts label. One day you ask the deli clerk for their nutrition information. She gives you a binder that contains information for all their prepared foods. You find that a 1/2 cup serving of the coleslaw contains 8 grams of carb, and a 1/2 cup serving of the baked beans contains 32 grams of carb. Since you buy these items regularly, you jot this information down so you can add it to your personal carb counting database when you get home.

When you get home, you measure out a 1/2 cup serving of each. The 1/2 cup of coleslaw looks like the amount you usually eat, but the 1/2 cup of beans looks small. You estimate that your typical serving of baked beans is closer to 3/4 cup. So you'll need to do some math to figure out the carb count in your serving of baked beans. Here's how:

32 g carb in 1/2 cup

1/4 is half of 1/2. So there are 16 g in a 1/4 cup of these beans (32 ÷ 2 = 16)

32 + 16 = 48

So, there are 48 grams of carb in a 3/4 cup serving of these baked beans. As we discussed in Chapter 5, you can add this information to your personal carb counting database so you'll have it for future reference.

Your eating style does not have to completely change because of carb counting; in fact, when you become skilled at carb counting, you may enjoy using convenience foods or some of your old recipes even more because you'll be able to predict how the meal will affect your blood glucose level.

Counting Carbs in Recipes

Just as you learned to estimate the nutrition information in prepared foods, you can also learn how to calculate the carbohydrate in servings from recipes.

Of course, you can avoid this exercise by using recipe books, cooking magazines, and food websites that provide nutrition information. All of the American Diabetes Association's recipes provide this information. In addition, most of the cookbooks and cooking magazines that are geared toward people with diabetes, people who want to lose weight, and people who are interested in healthier eating also provide carb counts for the recipes. This is a good way to get new recipes as well as learn about lower-calorie and lower-fat cooking techniques.

But there will always be cases where you want to figure out the carbs in a recipe that doesn't already provide nutritional information. It takes a little effort, but you just need to go through the exercise one time. Add your calculations to the recipe or to your database, and you'll have it handy for next time. Here's how to do it:

The How-To's of Recipe Carb Counting

Step 1

Gather the information and tools you'll need: the recipe, scratch paper, a pen or pencil, a calculator, and your favorite reference for carb counts. If this is an old family recipe without precise measurements, you'll need to come up with estimated amounts of each ingredient before starting.

Step 2

Go through the list of ingredients one by one and find each ingredient in your reference tools. Write down the grams of carb. Remember to make adjustments for the amount of the food used in the recipe (the amount used in the recipe may not match the default amount found in the book or on the website). For example, if the reference tool lists the carb count in 1 cup of flour and your recipe calls for 1/2 cup of flour, you'll have to divide the carb count in half.

Step 3

Add up the grams of carbohydrate from all the ingredients. This tells you the total grams of carbohydrate in the whole recipe.

Step 4

Divide the total carbohydrate grams by the number of servings. If this is a handwritten recipe, it may not tell you the number of servings—use your estimating skills.

Step 5

Write down the carb count per serving on the recipe or in your database of carb counts. Remember to also write down the number of servings or serving size you used for your calculation in Step 4.

Here's an example of how you can calculate a recipe's carbohydrate content. This is the ingredient list from a recipe for Moroccan chicken stew:

- 2 cups chicken broth
- 1/2 cup tomato paste
- 1 tsp ground cumin
- 1 tsp salt

- 1/4 tsp ground red pepper
- 1/8 tsp cinnamon
- 1/2 cup raisins
- 1 medium onion
- 1 Tbsp minced garlic
- 2 lb butternut squash
- 1 cup frozen peas
- 1 can (16 oz) chickpeas
- 4 chicken thighs

The recipe does not include nutritional information, but it does say that it feeds four people. We checked the database at nutrition.gov and recorded the following information:

Amount/Ingredients	Carbohydrate (g)
2 cups chicken broth	0
1/2 cup tomato paste	24
1 tsp ground cumin	0
1 tsp salt	0
1/4 tsp ground red pepper	0
1/8 tsp cinnamon	0
1/2 cup raisins	58
1 medium-size onion	8
1 Tbsp minced fresh garlic	4
2 lb butternut squash	52
1 cups frozen green peas	18
1 can (16 ounces) chickpeas	108
4 chicken thighs	0
Total grams of carbohydrate	**272**

So the entire pot of chicken stew made by this recipe totals 272 grams of carb. But you're not eating the whole pot! Remember, this recipe feeds four people.

So, each serving contains 68 grams of carbohydrate (272 ÷ 4) or about four and a half carb choices (68 ÷ 15).

Let's Review

Try to answer the following questions. Refer back to the chapter if you need help.

- What are two ways of figuring out the carb count of ready-to-eat foods that don't have a Nutrition Facts label? *Use data from a similar item; use an average of data from similar items*
- What are the steps for figuring out the carb count in recipes? *Find data on each ingredient; add it all up; divide by the number of servings*

Let's Practice

- Figure out the carb count in a few ready-to-eat foods you eat regularly using the averaging method.
- Figure out the carb count in an old family recipe. Remember to estimate the number of servings in the complete recipe.

Carb Counting Restaurant Meals and Takeout Food

The average American eats four or more restaurant meals each week. Many of us have hectic, busy lives, and eating out can be convenient and fun. If restaurant meals are part of the way you eat, this doesn't have to change once you start carb counting. With a little practice, you can learn to apply the principles of carb counting to just about any menu item at any restaurant.

Information for the Asking

Today, there's more nutrition information available for restaurant foods than ever before. Fast food restaurants like McDonald's, Burger King, and KFC post nutritional information in their restaurants and on their websites. Many national chains like Applebee's, Pizza Hut, and Panera Bread include nutritional information on their websites, and some include a "healthy" section on their menu, listing selections that are lower in fat and calories. Some also offer brochures or binders with nutrition information by request. If you often eat at these types of places, take a few minutes to visit their websites and look up the menu items you tend to order. Add this information to your personal database so you can access it easily next time.

Most small, independent restaurants do not have nutrition information readily available. This is true of fancy, special occasion restaurants as well as the mom-and-pop takeout place on the corner. When you eat in these types of restaurants, you'll need to do a little more work. Table 8.1 gives you an example of how you can keep a personal record of restaurant meals.

Tips to Make Your Best Guess

If you weigh and measure foods regularly at home, you'll be familiar with portion sizes. Remember to use these skills in restaurants, too. Measure portions by comparing them to your hands and common household items (refer back to the tips in Chapter 4, which can be particularly helpful in restaurants, where you don't have access to measuring spoons and cups or a food scale).

If the restaurant doesn't provide nutrition information, look for the same or a similar dish on the website of a national chain and use this information as a starting point for your estimation. For example, the nutrition information for chicken parmesan on the Macaroni Grill website can help you estimate the carb count in the chicken parmesan you get at your favorite local Italian place. To get even closer, check out the carb counts for the same dish at several different places and calculate an average.

If you ask, the restaurant staff may even be willing to share recipes with you so you can estimate the carb count based on the techniques covered in the last chapter.

Another helpful tactic is to order your favorite dishes for takeout so you can weigh and measure the portions at home. You can weigh the pieces of meat and bread, measure the servings of rice or pasta, and estimate the content of sauces and coatings. This exercise is usually quite eye-opening—restaurant portions are often very large! You may find that one meal can easily become two.

If you can't find information on some foods you regularly eat, see if you can find

If restaurant meals are part of the way you eat, this doesn't have to change once you start carb counting. With a little practice, you can learn to apply the principles of carb counting to just about any menu item at any restaurant.

Table 8.1 Sample Personal Database Record—Restaurant Meals

Meal	Serving (amount I eat)	Carbohydrate (g)
BURGER KING		
Original Whopper Jr. (no mayonnaise)	1	32
French fries	1/2 medium	23
Side garden salad	1	5
Salad dressing, Catalina	2 Tbsp	5
Total		**65**
LOCAL PIZZA PARLOR*		
12" cheese pizza with onions and mushrooms	3 slices	84
Total		**84**
LOCAL MEXICAN RESTAURANT†		
Fajitas	1 order (3 fajitas)	
Chicken and beef	4 oz	0
Grilled onions and peppers	2/3 cup	11
Tortillas, 6-inch	3	54
Guacamole	3 Tbsp	4
Tomatoes	1/2 cup	3
Rice, Mexican	1/3 cup	16
Refried beans	1/2 cup	20
Total		**108**

*Information accessed from Papa John's online nutritional calculator at http://www.papas-nutritional-calculator.com. Accessed 7 October 2018. †Based on the Nutrition Facts labels and nutrition information obtained from www.ars.usda.gov/nutrientdata (the U.S. Department of Agriculture searchable database). For more restaurant food nutrition information, see *The Diabetes Carbohydrate and Fat Gram Guide, 5th Edition* (2017), by Lea Ann Holzmeister.

a recipe for a similar dish on a recipe website, in a cookbook in the library, or in the collection of a friend or family member. Then use the recipe analysis techniques covered in Chapter 7. Don't forget sauces! They often contain added sugar, flour, or cornstarch, all of which contain carbohydrate and affect blood glucose. Here's a handy trick for estimating carb counts in sauces: add 5–10 grams of carbohydrate to your total to account for the "hidden" carbohydrate.

Restaurant Eating: Tips and Skills for Reducing Calories and Carbohydrates

One of the biggest problems with restaurant meals is that the portions are often huge. Here are tips and tactics to help you manage your portions and, as a result, carbs and calories:

- Avoid items on the menu that include words like large, giant, grande, supreme, extra-large, jumbo, double, triple, double-decker, king-size, monster, and super. Instead, choose items described as junior, single, petite, kiddie, and regular.
- If you see a weight for a piece of meat on the menu, it's most likely the raw weight. For example, you might see a hamburger referred to as a "quarter pound" of meat, a fillet weighing 6 ounces, or a slice of prime rib that weighs 10 ounces. Remember that these are averages, not exact weights, and that proteins lose weight in cooking. Refer to the box titled Raw to Cooked: Rules of Thumb in Chapter 4 to help you convert servings from raw weight to cooked weight.
- Consider ordering soup and salad, or an appetizer and a salad or soup. That may be enough for you. (See A Closer Look—Salad Bars for tips on choosing salads and soups—depending on the ingredients, they may not always be healthier options.)
- Ask for a half portion or share an entrée with another person.
- Ask for a takeout container at the beginning of the meal and place the extra food in it to take home.

A Note about Pizza

Pizza can be challenging for some people with diabetes. It can cause blood glucose to rise in some people, and it can cause a delayed rise in blood glucose in other people. For starters, when you eat pizza, do your best to get a solid carb count. Use some of the techniques described in this chapter: check the websites of national chains and take an average of the carb counts you find for similar types of pizza. If you use a blood glucose meter (more about that in Chapter 9), you can check your blood glucose 2 hours after you eat to see how the pizza affected you. If there is a lot of meat and cheese on the pizza and/or if your 2-hour blood glucose wasn't what you expected, check your blood glucose again 3–5 hours after starting the meal. If your blood glucose is high, then the high fat content in the pizza could have been the cause. Keep close records the next time you eat pizza, too. This is important information to know—and you'll use it every time you eat pizza.

A Closer Look—Salad Bars

It's easy to lose track of your carbohydrate targets when you're eating out. Menu choices that seem "light" can often have lots of hidden carbohydrate. Let's say you go out to lunch and have soup and a salad from the salad bar. That sounds like a good choice—but it all depends on what you put on your salad and what type of soup you have.

The so-called "light" lunch represented in Table 8.2 can easily put you way above your carb target. How can you bring down the carb count of this meal? Here are some suggestions:

- Reduce the amount of croutons to 1/2 cup and save 8 grams of carbohydrate.
- Reduce the salad dressing to 1 Tbsp and save 12 grams of carbohydrate.

Table 8.2 A So-Called "Light Lunch"

Food	Carbohydrate (g)
3 cups salad greens	8
Bacon bits, egg, ham	0
1/3 cup kidney beans	15
1/3 cup chickpeas	15
1 cup croutons	15
1/3 cup fat-free salad dressing	15
1 1/2 cups chicken noodle soup	30
Total carbohydrate	**98, or 6 1/2 carb choices**

- Combine the kidney and chickpeas in a 1/3 cup serving and save 15 grams of carbohydrate.
- Only have 1 cup of the soup and save 10 grams of carbohydrate.

With these changes, your total savings is 45 grams of carbohydrate, and you're back in range without giving up too much flavor or quantity of food.

Case Study: Meet John

John worked at the mall and ate all his lunches at the food court during the workweek. He rotated his choices from the various ethnic cafes and generally ordered the same item each time. He was trying to eat 60–75 grams of carbohydrate at lunch, but he had no idea how many grams of carb were in his lunch choices. So his diabetes care provider suggested that he bring home each of his regular food court meals to measure and record their carb counts. Here's what he found.

Lunch #1: Vegetable stir-fry with fried rice

2 1/2 cups of fried rice = 105 grams carbohydrate
1 1/2 cups stir-fried vegetables = 15 grams carbohydrate
Sauce = 10 grams carbohydrate

This meal had 130 grams of carbohydrate, which was nearly twice as much as John's target for lunch.

Lunch #2: Beef enchiladas

2 small beef enchiladas = 35 grams carbohydrate

It was difficult to assess the individual ingredients and amounts in this meal. So John weighed the enchiladas and looked up nutritional information for similarly sizes beef enchiladas on several restaurant websites. After taking an average of that information, he figured the meal had 35 grams of carbohydrate. This was much less than his lunchtime target of 60–75 grams.

Lunch #3: A gyro sandwich with cucumber salad

2 ounces pita bread = 30 grams carbohydrate
4 ounces lamb = 0 grams carbohydrate
1 cup cucumbers mixed with 1/3 cup yogurt = 5 grams carbohydrate

The total for this meal was 35 grams of carbohydrate, much below his target of 60–75 grams.

Lunch #4: Sushi and miso soup

1 Maki roll with seafood and vegetables (six pieces) = 48 grams carbohydrate
1 cup miso soup = 8 grams carbohydrate

Sushi can be difficult to carb count because there are many different kinds and varieties in preparation. The majority of carbohydrate in sushi comes from the rice. John looked up sushi rolls' nutritional information on several websites and took an average. He decided that six pieces of Maki roll totaled about 48 grams of carb. That total plus the miso soup total put John within his target range.

Lunch #5: Deep-dish pizza with sausage and extra cheese and a garden salad with honey mustard dressing

2 slices pizza = 74 grams carbohydrate
Small garden salad = 2 grams carbohydrate
2 Tbsp honey mustard dressing = 6 grams carbohydrate

John knew that the slices were from a 14-inch pizza. By checking several websites and taking an average, he estimated that each slice of the pizza had 37 grams of carbohydrate, and he was eating two large slices. The pizza alone contained about 74 grams of carbohydrate.

This exercise was very useful to John and his CDE. It helped John learn more about some of his favorite meals and how they affected his blood glucose. It helped his CDE learn more about John's food preferences and eating habits. Together, they used the information to refine his carb goals, his eating plan, and his blood glucose targets. His CDE suggested some simple changes to the meals that would make a big difference in his post-meal blood glucose. For example, she suggested that ordering two medium-size pieces of the pizza in the future or choosing a thin-crust pizza with some non-starchy veggies, such as mushrooms, peppers, and onions, would lower the total calories and fat in addition to carb grams.

Let's Review

Try to answer the following questions. Refer back to the chapter if you need help.

- What are two different ways you can figure out a carb count estimate for a favorite restaurant meal when nutritional information is not provided on the menu or website? *Use data from the same menu item from a different restaurant; order it for takeout and weigh and measure at home*

- What are two ways you can manage your portion sizes when eating out at a restaurant? *Share a dish with someone else; take half of it home for another meal*

Let's Practice

Use your new knowledge to work through the following exercises.

- Pick one of your favorite meals from a casual restaurant that includes nutritional information on its website. Create a database entry for the meal like the examples in Table 8.1, including drinks, sides, and condiments. Any surprises? How does it compare to your carb target for the meal? What changes could you make to the meal to make it work better with your eating plan?
- Bring home one of your favorite takeout/delivery meals from a local place that doesn't provide nutritional information. Before eating, separate out the components of the meal and measure them. Write down the foods and the amounts of each part of the meal. Use your favorite carb counting resource to look up the carb count in each one, and add up the total. Any surprises? How does it compare to your carb target for the meal? What changes could you make to the meal to make it work better with your eating plan?

9

Blood Glucose Pattern Management: Fine-Tuning Your Plan

You've learned how to identify carbohydrate in the foods you eat, how to measure how much carb you're eating, and how to add it all up. Now what do you do with all this information?

The next step is what diabetes care providers call "pattern management." Pattern management is a way to use your records to learn how your body reacts to a variety of factors and then adjust your diabetes plan and your daily activities to consistently get to your blood glucose goals. Your pattern management data can also provide valuable information to your diabetes care provider, who can use this information to make adjustments to your care plan and help you learn more about diabetes self-management.

Keep in mind, there is no such thing as "perfect" blood glucose management. Let's face it—there's no such thing as perfect anything! There are just too many things that can influence your blood glucose, and life is too unpredictable. However, you certainly *can* minimize the ups and downs—and as a result, keep yourself healthy today and for years to come. The best way to do that is to learn from your own experiences so you can better predict how your body will react to different foods, activities, and situations.

A Note about Pattern Management

It's important to note that pattern management requires the use of a blood glucose monitoring device. If you have prediabetes, or have just been diagnosed with type 2 diabetes, you might not be using a device yet. There are two types of blood glucose monitoring devices: the traditional blood glucose meter, used to draw a tiny amount of blood from your finger to check blood glucose levels, and the newer continuous glucose monitors, which are wearable devices that are programmed to check your blood glucose at certain times of the day. (You may hear people refer to this method as CGM, which stands for continuous glucose monitoring.) There are new advances in blood glucose monitoring technology all the time. The latest breakthrough as of this writing is a CGM touchscreen device that you can use to scan a small sensor attached to your body.

Pattern management requires use of a blood glucose meter. If you are not using either a manual or a continuous blood glucose meter, talk to your diabetes care provider about whether it makes sense to add this tool to your care plan.

Regardless of the device you use, capturing your blood glucose reading several times a day allows you to see how your blood glucose levels respond to food, exercise, stress, and other factors. Most people check their blood glucose two to three times a day, on a rotating schedule. Common times to check blood glucose are first thing after waking (often called the "fasting" reading), 1–2 hours after a meal, right before eating a meal, and right before going to bed. For example, on Monday, you might do a check when you wake up and 2 hours after eating breakfast. On Tuesday, you check before lunch and 2 hours after lunch. Rotating like this allows you to get a variety of readings at different times and under different conditions. If you're not using a blood glucose monitoring device, talk to your diabetes care provider about whether a device makes sense for you.

Understanding Hyperglycemia and Hypoglycemia

You've probably heard or read the terms *hyperglycemia* and *hypoglycemia*. As a person with diabetes, it is important for you to understand what they mean, how to recognize them if they happen, and what to do about them.

Glycemia refers to blood glucose, the level of sugar in your blood. *Hyper-* means high, and *hypo-* means low. So at the most basic level, *hyperglycemia* means high blood sugar and *hypoglycemia* means low blood sugar. But in both cases, the terms are used when levels are dangerously high or low. Both can have serious effects on your health.

Hyperglycemia is defined as blood glucose levels at or above 200 mg/dL. You may remember that for most people, the high end of the target range for blood glucose after meals is 180 mg/dL. So as you can see, blood glucose levels have to be seriously elevated to qualify as hyperglycemia.

The same goes for *hypoglycemia*, which is defined as blood glucose levels at or below 70 mg/dL. If blood glucose levels fall lower than 54 mg/dL, the hypoglycemia is considered clinically significant and requires immediate medical attention.

Pattern management can help prevent both hyperglycemia and hypoglycemia. We'll talk more about both conditions in Chapter 10, when we talk about medications that lower blood glucose.

Pattern Management: It Takes Three Steps

In Chapter 5, you learned how to track the amount of carbohydrate in the meals and snacks you eat each day. Pattern management builds on that basic skill, by adding your blood glucose meter readings and medication information to your food logs so you can see the relationship between what you eat, the medicines you take, and your blood glucose levels.

Some blood glucose meters can identify and report patterns, and all of the new CGM devices have this capability. There are also pattern management smartphone apps that can help. But you may still find it helpful to capture and review your patterns the old-fashioned way while you're learning. Follow these steps.

Pattern management adds your blood glucose meter readings and medication information to your food logs so you can see the relationship between what you eat, the medicines you take, and your blood glucose levels.

....

Step 1: Find the Patterns

Gather up a few weeks' worth of blood glucose records. You'll want to have at least two readings on each day. Write your blood glucose targets at the top of the record sheet for easy reference.

> *Note:* Remember, there is no one-size-fits-all target for blood glucose. Your diabetes care provider will help you set goals that are right for you. On average, the before-meal target is between 80 and 130 mg/dL and the after-meal target (1–2 hours after beginning to eat) is less than 180 mg/dL.

Use one colored marker, pen, or highlighter to circle all the blood glucose readings in your records that are *above* your target. Then use a different colored pen to circle all those that are *below* your target.

Step 2: Observe the Patterns

Now look for patterns in your highs and lows. If you have food logs for those weeks, that's great—look for connections between what and when you ate and your blood glucose levels. However, if you don't have complete food logs, that's OK; you can still look for patterns in the times and days of the week of your highs and lows. By looking at a calendar, you may be able to connect high or low records with a special event or a particularly stressful day.

Here are some things to consider:
- If many of your blood glucose results are *above* your target range, consider whether one or several of the following could be the cause:
  - Too much carbohydrate at meals
  - Less physical activity than planned
  - Physical or emotional stress

- ◆ If you take blood glucose–lowering medication, you may need an increased dose or need additional or different medications. Check with your diabetes care provider.
- If many of your blood glucose values are *below* your target range, consider whether one or several of the following could be the cause:
  - ◆ Delayed or missed meals or snacks
  - ◆ Physical activity
  - ◆ Too little carbohydrate at meals or snacks
  - ◆ If you take blood glucose–lowering medication (including insulin) you may need help with your dose or need an adjustment. Check with your diabetes care provider.

Also look for patterns in when the highs and lows happen. Are they often first thing in the morning, when you wake up? Do they often happen on the weekends, when you might not be following your eating plan as closely? This type of information can be very useful as you fine-tune your plan.

Step 3: Plan and Take Action

After you've identified patterns, plan a course of action to limit these situations in the future. Sometimes a simple change, like adjusting your eating plan, is enough. For example, you may find that a couple of hours after dinner, your blood glucose is usually higher than your target. When you look at your food logs, you see that you're eating several carbohydrate choices at dinner. Therefore, a logical action would be to reduce the number of carbohydrate choices in your evening meal and then check your blood glucose a few evenings to determine whether this change has brought your blood glucose levels into your target range.

Note: If your blood glucose results are consistently at or above 200 mg/dL (hyperglycemia) or below 70 mg/dL (hypoglycemia), don't wait—contact or make an appointment with your diabetes care provider to get help adjusting your diabetes plan.

As you go through this exercise, you may begin to appreciate the value of keeping track of more details in your daily logs. As your personal carb counting database

What Else Can Affect Blood Glucose?

There are many factors that can affect your blood glucose. As you move into pattern management, you may want to consider adding some or all of the following information into your recordkeeping:

Physical Activity

Being physically active generally lowers blood glucose. Being physically active is an important part of managing your diabetes and an important part of staying healthy. If you're not already physically active, it's always a good idea to start. Any amount of activity is good—but it's a good idea to check with your health care team before beginning a new exercise regimen. When you are physically active, note the type of activity, how long you did it, and the time of day in your records.

Emotions, Stress, Illness, and Unusual Situations

Changes in day-to-day events can affect blood glucose, too. When you are ill or a loved one is ill, when you're dealing with a deadline at work, or when you're having conflict in a relationship, you may see changes in your results. It's important to record information about the emotions you're feeling and the stressful situations you're dealing with. It's also important to record positive emotions and situations. For example, vacations may be a positive change to your regular routine, but vacations can also cause you to eat differently and at different times. Women can note menstrual periods in their records as well; the various phases of the menstrual cycle, including the hormonal surges of adolescence and menopause, can affect blood glucose trends.

Medications

If you take blood glucose–lowering medications, it's important to track the medications you take, how much, and when. This information, along with all the other factors in your records, will help fine-tune your diabetes management. For more information about carb counting while taking blood glucose–lowering medications, see Chapter 10.

Most people find it easier to keep one record that includes space for all of the factors that affect blood glucose. There are a variety of tools available, from paper-based systems to smartphone apps and websites. Appendix 2 includes a list of tools that may be helpful.

grows, this will become easier—you'll already know the carb counts of your regular meals and snacks, and the effects of your regular activities and exercise routines.

Using Technology for Pattern Management

As with many things in our world, technology has revolutionized blood glucose management capabilities. Of course, you can still keep pen-and-paper records of your blood glucose readings if you like. But once you learn more about the available technology, you may appreciate the convenience it offers.

One of the main benefits of new blood glucose monitoring technology is the ability of the devices to transmit data to another device for storage. Different brands of blood glucose monitors do this in different ways. Some transmit data to your computer or other device via Bluetooth technology, some send data to "the cloud" so information can be accessed remotely by your diabetes care provider, and some allow you to plug the meter into your computer via a USB port to download the data. Some brands provide a smartphone app you can download to help you record readings on the go. (See the box Choosing a Blood Glucose Meter for more information.)

Choosing a Blood Glucose Meter

There are many different blood glucose meters on the market, with a variety of bells and whistles. When choosing a meter, you'll want to consider ease of use, size and shape, accuracy and compatibility with your computer, smartphone, and other devices. But before you get too far into comparing models, you'll want to know what your health insurance policy covers. The meters themselves are fairly affordable (typically between $10 and $50); the expense comes from the test strips, which can cost anywhere from 50 cents to $2 per strip, depending on the type of meter. Insurance providers often name a "preferred" meter and test strip brand that they will cover at a higher level. Of course, you can always choose a different model, but you'll have to pay more out of pocket for the meter and its strips.

Be sure to talk to your diabetes care provider about your test strip expenses. If cost is an issue, your testing schedule can be adjusted to help you get the most impactful data for the lowest cost.

Case Study: Meet Roberta

Let's look at how pattern management works with a practical example.

Roberta was diagnosed with type 2 diabetes 8 years ago. She uses a blood glucose meter and practices carb counting. She's been pretty successful managing her blood glucose levels. Her target blood glucose goals are:

- Fasting and before meals: 120 mg/dL
- 2 hours after meals: 190 mg/dL

Over the past years, Roberta's blood glucose has been creeping up. And recently, Roberta has started feeling tired and sometimes experiencing blurry vision. Her diabetes care provider suggested that she follow the pattern management steps for a few weeks to get back on track and see if her care plan needed adjustment.

Step 1: Find the Patterns

Roberta kept detailed records for 2 weeks. She went through her records and circled the high readings in red. She found that all of her readings were occasionally higher than her target, but that the after-dinner and fasting blood glucose levels were consistently high.

Step 2: Observe the Patterns

Roberta compared her blood glucose readings to her food logs and looked for patterns. She could see a connection between the amount of carb she ate at a meal and the high readings after. She also saw that she was regularly exceeding her carbohydrate goals at dinner. On a positive note, Roberta noticed that her after-dinner readings were lower when she took a 30-minute walk before she ate.

Step 3: Plan and Take Action

Roberta renewed her carb counting efforts at all meals, with special focus on dinner. She eliminated the bread basket from the table and reduced her serving sizes of rice and potatoes to get her dinner meals back within her carb counting goals. She also made sure to get in her 30-minute walk before dinner each day. Soon Roberta's blood glucose was back in her target range, and she could feel the difference in her energy level and her vision.

Don't Check a Lot, Check Smart

Hopefully Roberta's example helps you understand the value of recordkeeping and pattern management. Remember, the details will be different for each person. Your blood glucose–monitoring schedule will vary, depending on your goals, care plan, the device you use, and your insurance coverage. No matter when or how often you check your blood glucose level, keep in mind that you want to check smart versus checking a lot. Checking smart means checking strategically. Always have in mind why and what you are checking and what information this check will provide. Pattern management is an investment of time and energy, but it can pay big dividends in how you feel day-to-day and for your long-term health.

Let's Review

- What is pattern management? *Tracking patterns in your blood glucose level in relation to foods, activity levels, stress, time of day, etc.*
- What are upper and lower blood glucose readings that should trigger an immediate call to your diabetes care provider? *Under 54 mg/dL; above 200 mg/dL*
- What factors should you consider in choosing a blood glucose meter? *What your insurance will cover; cost; accuracy; cost of supplies; convenience*

Let's Practice

Use your new knowledge and skills to work through these exercises.

- If you use a blood glucose–monitoring device, look at 1 week's worth of readings. Note the readings that are higher and lower than your goal. Do you see patterns in high or low readings related to the time of day, or your activity or stress level that day? What could you do differently to minimize those highs and lows?
- If you have food logs for the same week, compare the readings to your meals. Do you see a relationship between high or low readings and what you ate? What could you do differently to minimize those highs and lows?

10

Insulin and Other Blood Glucose–Lowering Medications

All people with type 1 diabetes take insulin, because their bodies do not produce any insulin on their own. But if you have prediabetes or have just been diagnosed with type 2 diabetes, you may not take any diabetes medications at all. However, because of the progressive nature of type 2 diabetes, most people with type 2 will eventually require some type of medication. In fact, most people with type 2 diabetes will eventually take some form of insulin to manage their blood glucose levels.

Some people with type 2 diabetes have reservations about taking diabetes medication and taking insulin in particular. They may think that needing insulin to manage their type 2 diabetes means that they "failed" in their efforts to manage their blood glucose with diet and exercise. Please know that this is not true!

We now know that type 2 diabetes is a progressive disease, which means that the way it affects the body changes over time. Treatments that are effective in year one may not work in year five, and so on. These changes are not anyone's fault; they are simply the nature of the disease. Over the years, you'll work with your diabetes care provider to adjust your care plan to meet your changing needs. Resources like this book can help you be prepared now and into the future.

Scientists now know that type 2 diabetes is a progressive disease, which means that the way it affects the body changes over time. What works in year one may not work in year five, and so on. These changes are not anyone's fault; there are simply the nature of the disease.

Carb counting is compatible with all the different types of diabetes medication. However, the way you *use* carb counting may vary depending on your medication plan. We'll explain more as we go through this chapter.

Types of Diabetes Medications

There are two main categories of diabetes medications: oral and injectable. Oral medications are pills that you take by mouth. Injectable medications are injected under the skin using a needle and syringe, a continuous pump, or a device called a pen. Within each category, there are different types of medications that work in different ways.

But there are new types of medication and new delivery methods being introduced all the time. For example, there is now a new type of insulin that you breathe in through a device like an asthma inhaler. Your diabetes care provider will work with you to choose a medication regimen that best suits your preferences, goals, and insurance coverage and will make adjustments as the disease progresses.

People with type 1 diabetes *must* take some form of insulin, because their bodies do not produce insulin on their own. However, people with type 2 diabetes have a wide variety of diabetes medications from which to choose to help manage their blood glucose levels. For most people with type 2 diabetes, their medication regimen will change over the years. Many people may start with one oral medication and then add one or two other types of non-insulin medication. And, eventually, they begin to use insulin. Some even take insulin in combination with another medication.

Oral Medications

Take a look at Table 10.1. The table lists all of the oral diabetes medications on the market today.

Table 10.1 Oral Diabetes Medications

Drug class	Generic name (brand name)	How do they work?	Can they cause hypoglycemia?
Sulfonylureas	glipizide (Glucotrol and Glucotrol XL); glyburide (Micronase, Glynase, Diabeta); glimepiride (Amaryl)	Stimulate the pancreas to release more insulin	Yes
Meglitinides	repaglinide (Prandin); nateglinide (Starlix)	Stimulate the pancreas to release more insulin	Yes
Biguanides	metformin (Glucophage, Glucophase XR, Glumetza, Fortamet)	Decreases amount of glucose produced by the liver; helps muscle tissue absorb glucose	No
Thiazolidinediones (TZDs) (sometimes called glitazones)	pioglitazone (Actos)	Helps insulin work better in muscles and fat; decreases amount of glucose produced by the liver	No
α-Glucosidase inhibitors	acarbose (Precose); miglitol (Glyset)	Blocks breakdown of starches in the intestine; slows the breakdown of some sugars	No
DPP-4 inhibitors	sitagliptin (Januvia); saxagliptin (Onglyza); linagliptin (Tradjenta); alogliptin (Nesina)	Prolongs action of GLP-1, a natural compound that helps lower blood glucose	No
Bile acid sequestrants (BASs)	colesevelam (Welchol)	Unclear; helps remove cholesterol from the body	No
SGLT2 inhibitors	canagliflozin (Invokana); dapagliflozin (Farxiga); empagliflozin (Jardiance)	Blocks absorption of glucose in the kidneys	No
Dopamine-2 agonists	bromocriptine quick release (Cycloset)	Helps lower blood glucose levels after a meal	Yes

Source: *Diabetes Forecast Consumer Guide 2018.*

> *You should not adjust your dose of oral diabetes medications on your own. If you have questions about your dosage, talk with your diabetes care provider.*
> ....

The most common oral medication for people with type 2 diabetes is metformin. Many people begin taking metformin right after being diagnosed. Some people take a combination of metformin and other oral medications or insulin to manage their blood glucose levels.

All of these oral medications are taken in a fixed dose. You should not adjust your dose of oral diabetes medications on your own. If you have questions about your dosage, talk with your diabetes care provider.

Injectable Medications

In addition to the many forms of insulin, there are two other kinds of injectable medication that can help people with diabetes manage their blood glucose. Table 10.2 shows the three different classes of injectable diabetes medications.

Non-insulin injectables

There are two types of non-insulin injectable medications for diabetes: the amylin analog and the GLP-1 receptor agonist. The amylin analog, pramlintide, can be used by people with type 1 or type 2 diabetes. Drugs in the GLP-1 receptor agonist class can be used alone or with insulin, for people with type 1 or type 2 diabetes. Some drugs in this class, like Trulicity and Bydureon, are taken once a week. Victoza is taken daily, and Byetta is taken twice a day.

Insulin

While insulin has been used for decades, there have been many advancements in recent years that make insulin more convenient and easier to use. There are now some insulin formulations that can work for as long as 42 hours, and there are pumps and pens that make it easier to get your insulin dose. Now there's even an insulin you can breathe in through an inhaling device!

Insulin is classified by how quickly or how long it works in the body. You'll hear insulin referred to as rapid-acting, short-acting, intermediate-acting, and long-acting. These terms refer to how long it takes for the medicine to have an effect on blood glucose and how long the effect lasts. There are also "premixed"

Table 10.2 Injectable Medications for Diabetes

Drug class	Generic name (brand name)	How do they work?	Can they cause hypoglycemia?
Amylin analog	pramlintide (Symlin)	Used with mealtime insulin to slow the digestion of food in the stomach; reduces glucose production in the liver	No
GLP-1 receptor agonists (sometimes called incretin mimetics)	exenatide (Byetta); liraglutide (Victoza); albiglutide (Tanzeum); dulaglutide (Trulicity); exenatide (Byetta); exenatide extended release (Bydureon); liraglutide (Victoza); albiglutide (Eperzan, Tanzeum); lixisenatide (Adlyxin); semaglutide (Ozempic)	Can be used alone or with insulin; slows glucose absorption in the gut; increases insulin production (type 2 only); decreases glucose production in the liver	No
Insulin	lispro (Humalog); aspart (Novolog); glulisine (Apidra); NPH (isophane); glargine (Lantus); detemir (Levemir); degludec (Tresiba); glargine (Toujeo)	Facilitates glucose absorption by the body's cells	Yes
Insulin plus GLP-1 receptor agonists	Glargine/lixisenatide (Soliqua); degludec/liraglutide (Xultophy)	Helps release insulin when blood glucose is high and helps glucose enter the cells	Low risk

Source: *Diabetes Forecast Consumer Guide 2018.*

insulin formulas that combine an intermediate-acting insulin with a short-acting insulin in one dose. Table 10.3 shows different types of insulin and the timing of their activity.

Can I Adjust My Insulin Dose on My Own?

You can learn to adjust your insulin dose based on what you eat, your activity level, and other factors, like guidance from a certified diabetes educator (CDE). This is not required; it is a personal decision based on your comfort level. If you're interested in learning more about self-adjusting insulin doses, talk with your diabetes care provider about how it might work for you. Many people use advanced carb counting methods to help them adjust their insulin doses. We'll talk more about how to do this in Chapter 11. But remember, you should always talk to your diabetes care provider before using these techniques.

Insulin Delivery Methods

Insulin cannot be taken in pill form, because it is broken down by digestive enzymes. Traditionally, insulin has been delivered through *subcutaneous injection,* meaning it is injected under the skin into a layer of fat. As mentioned above, there is a new type of insulin that can be delivered via a device similar to an asthma inhaler. In the future, it is likely that researchers will discover other insulin delivery methods. But for now, injection is still the most common way to take insulin. There are three current methods used to inject insulin: a regular syringe injection, an insulin pen, or a pump. Let's look at each separately.

Syringe Injection

Syringes are disposable and come in many sizes, and the needles come in a variety of thicknesses and lengths. They can be used to directly inject insulin under the skin.

People new to insulin often express fear of needles or concern about the pain of injections. Because insulin needs to be injected into an area that has a layer of fat under the skin, the pain is minimal. (Common spots for injections are the stomach, hips, thighs, buttocks, and back of the arms, all of which have few nerve endings.) Also, people who inject insulin directly follow a schedule of rotating injection sites so no one area gets injected too often. If you plan to inject insulin, talk to your diabetes care provider about the best way to manage your injection routine.

Table 10.3 The Action of Insulins

Insulin (brand name)	Onset	Peak	Duration
RAPID-ACTING			
Lispro (Humalog)	10–20 minutes	30–90 minutes	3–5 hours
Aspart (Fiasp)	2.5 minutes	50–70 minutes	About 5 hours
Aspart (Novolog)	10–20 minutes	40–50 minutes	3–5 hours
Glulisine (Apidra)	10–20 minutes	30–90 minutes	2–4 hours
Inhaled insulin powder (Afreeze)	3–7 minutes	12–15 minutes	1.5–3 hours
SHORT-ACTING			
Regular insulin or Novolin	30–60 minutes	1.5–2 hours	Up to 8 hours
Regular Humulin	30–60 minutes	2–4 hours	5–8 hours
INTERMEDIATE-ACTING			
NPH (Novolin N)	90 minutes	4–12 hours	Up to 24 hour
NPH (Humulin N)	1–3 hours	8 hours	12–16 hours
LONG-ACTING (BASAL)			
Glargine (Basaglar, Lantus)	1 hour	No peak time; insulin is delivered at a steady level	24 hours
Detemir (Levemir)	1.5 hours	6–8 hours	Up to 24 hours
ULTRA-LONG-ACTING			
Degludec (Tresiba)	1 hour	No peak time	At least 42 hours
Glargine (Toujeo)	6 hours	No peak	36 hours
PREMIXED*			
Humulin 70/30	30–60 minutes	Varies	12–16 hours
Novolin 70/30	30 minutes	Varies	Up to 24 hours
Novolog 70/30	10–20 minutes	Varies	Up to 24 hours
Humulin 50/50	10–15 minutes	Varies	16–22 hours
Humalog mix 75/25	10–15 minutes	Varies	16–22 hours

*Premixed insulins combine an intermediate-acting insulin with a short-acting insulin. The numbers after the name show the proportions of the two types in the dose; for example, Humulin 70/30 contains 70% intermediate-acting insulin and 30% short-acting insulin. The first number always represents the intermediate-acting insulin. Source: *Diabetes Forecast Consumer Guide 2018*.

Insulin Pumps

Today, more and more people are choosing to use an insulin pump. Many find that an insulin pump gives them greater flexibility in managing their diabetes and helps them improve their blood glucose management. Pumps are generally not used by people new to insulin therapy, but they are a convenient option for people with more insulin experience. Pumps aim to mimic the action of a healthy pancreas, by delivering small steady doses of insulin throughout the day and larger doses with meals.

There are three main types of insulin pumps, and new technology is being introduced all the time. The first type, sometimes called the traditional insulin pump, consists of a battery-powered pump and an insulin reservoir. The pump delivers insulin through a thin plastic tube called a *cannula*, which is inserted into your skin with a small needle. The cannula remains inserted into your body, and you carry the device in your pocket or a belt holster.

The second type is a tubeless system. These are sometimes called "patch pumps." They contain the same parts as a traditional pump, but the reservoir, pump, and cannula are all contained in one case without tubing. The device is attached to your body via a self-adhesive strip and replaced every 3 days. The cannula is automatically inserted after the device is attached to the skin. A separate unattached device, similar to a pager, is used to program the pump to provide insulin doses throughout the day.

The third, and newest, type of insulin pump is called a hybrid-closed loop and sensor augmented pump. This new type of pump combines an insulin pump with a continuous blood glucose monitoring sensor, allowing the pump to adjust basal or background insulin doses based on current blood glucose levels. This type of device requires carb counting skills, because you must enter your planned carb intake into the device before meals.

If you are interested in using an insulin pump, talk with your diabetes care provider. You'll also want to consider the factors listed in Which Insulin Delivery Method Should I Choose? on page 93.

Insulin Pens

Many people prefer insulin pens to syringes because they find them to be more accurate, easier to use, and easier to transport than syringes. Insulin pens get their name because they are about the size and shape of a pen, but they are filled with insulin instead of ink. They also include a dial that can be adjusted to select your dose. To use, you attach a small needle (as with syringes, pen needles come in a variety of widths and lengths), dial your dose, and inject into your chosen site. Pens are available in "pre-filled" disposable versions that deliver insulin in single-unit doses and in "durable" or "permanent" versions, which require the insertion of an insulin cartridge and can be used again and again.

Which Insulin Delivery Method Should I Choose?

Choosing an insulin delivery method is an important decision. Here are some factors to consider:

- *What does your health insurance cover?* Devices and supplies can get expensive, especially since you'll be using them frequently, every day of the year. Check with your health insurance provider to see what type of diabetes devices and supplies are covered and at what rates. When comparing costs, remember to figure out the volume of supplies you'll need each day, month, and year and calculate the expense accordingly.
- *What does my diabetes care team recommend?* Your diabetes care team is a great resource when making this decision. They most likely have experience with many different kinds of devices, they know your care plan, and they probably have a good sense of your self-management style.
- *Do you have physical limitations that may influence your choice?* If you have vision problems, you may have difficulty reading the measurement lines on a syringe. If you have dexterity problems, you may find injections difficult. There are tools to help with these types of challenges, if you are limited in your choice of device. But if you have the freedom to choose among the three delivery methods, these are things to consider.

Know Your Medications

It is important that you know the type of blood glucose–lowering medication(s) you take, when to take each one, how they work to help manage blood glucose, and how the medication works in conjunction with the carbohydrate you eat to control your blood glucose. Talk with your diabetes care provider to make sure you have all of the information you need. Be sure to record the type, dose, and timing of each medication daily. You can record it along with your blood glucose results and your food diary, or you may use another form. (Refer to Chapter 5 for more information on recordkeeping.) Whatever method you choose, this information will help you and your diabetes care providers interpret your blood glucose results and customize your care plan.

What about Hypoglycemia?

These medications are very effective at lowering blood glucose. But you can get too much of a good thing! Some medications may cause blood glucose to drop too low if you don't eat enough carbohydrate or don't account for other changes in your routine (see Tables 10.1 and 10.2). This is why carb counting and pattern management are so important for people who take diabetes medications, especially the types that can cause hypoglycemia.

Studies have shown that the most serious risk for hypoglycemia is for people with type 1 diabetes. However, anyone who takes a medication that can cause hypoglycemia should be aware of the condition, how to prevent it, how to recognize it, and how to treat it if it occurs.

Symptoms of Hypoglycemia

If you take one of these medications, you should familiarize yourself with the symptoms and treatments for hypoglycemia. Some people can have hypoglycemia without experiencing any symptoms. However, most people experience one or more of the following:

- Shakiness
- Dizziness
- Sweating
- Hunger
- Headache
- Pale skin color
- Sudden moodiness or behavior changes, such as crying for no apparent reason
- Clumsiness or jerky movements
- Seizure
- Difficulty paying attention or confusion

- Tingling sensations around the mouth
- Heart pounding sensation

The only way to know for sure if you are experiencing hypoglycemia is to check your blood glucose. Remember, blood glucose levels at or below 70 mg/dL qualify as hypoglycemia, and levels below 54 mg/dL require immediate medical attention.

> *The only way to know for sure if you are experiencing hypoglycemia is to check your blood glucose.*

Other Medications Can Cause Hypoglycemia, Too

It's important to note that there are some medications prescribed for other conditions that can contribute to hypoglycemia. For example, β-blockers, a common class of drugs often used to treat high blood pressure, can lower blood glucose levels and mask symptoms of hypoglycemia. It is very important that your diabetes care provider know about every prescription and over-the-counter medicine that you take.

How to Treat Hypoglycemia

Even when you are consciously trying to prevent hypoglycemia, it can surprise you. Therefore, you need to be ready to deal with it quickly, if it happens. If you are experiencing symptoms of hypoglycemia, check your blood glucose right away if possible. If your blood glucose level is below 54 mg/dL, seek medical attention immediately. If it is below 70 mg/dL but above 54 mg/dL, remember the Rule of 15: eat something with about 15 grams of carbohydrate and then wait 15 minutes. After the 15 minutes is up, check your blood glucose level. If it is still less than 70 md/dL, repeat the steps.

Note: In cases of severe hypoglycemia, you may receive an injection of a drug called glucagon. Glucagon is a hormone produced in the pancreas that stimulates your liver to release stored glucose into your bloodstream when your blood glucose levels are too low. Some people with diabetes keep glucagon in an emergency kit to be used in case of severe hypoglycemia. Talk to your diabetes care provider to see if a glucagon prescription makes sense for you.

Back in Chapter 2, you learned that one carb "choice" contains 15 grams of carb and read examples of a few food servings that contain that amount of carbohydrate. However, you won't necessarily have ready access to a small apple or a glass of orange juice when you're experiencing symptoms of hypoglycemia. For that reason, many people with diabetes carry glucose tablets or gel with them just in case. Brands of glucose tablets and gels can vary; check the label for instructions. Usually, each glucose tablet contains 4–5 grams of carb, so you'd take three to four tablets to treat hypoglycemia. Glucose tablets and gels work best because they raise your blood glucose quickly. Plus, they're convenient and easy to store. Other options include 10–15 jelly beans, 4–6 ounces of fruit juice, or 4–6 ounces of soda (not diet soda; remember, artificial sweeteners do not contain carbohydrate).

Follow the Rule of 15 to Treat Symptoms of Hypoglycemia
- Check blood glucose. If it is below 70 mg/dL:
  - Eat 15 grams of carbohydrate.
  - Wait 15 minutes.
  - Check your blood glucose.
  - If your reading is at or below 70 mg/dL, repeat these steps.

Convenient Sources of 15 Grams of Carbohydrate
- Three to four glucose tablets, depending on the brand (each has 4–5 grams of carbohydrate)
- Glucose gel or other preparations of pure glucose
- 4–6 ounces of fruit juice (any type)
- 4–6 ounces regular soda (not diet)
- 10–15 jelly beans

Places to Store Glucose Tablets or Gels
- In your bag or pocket
- In your car's glove compartment
- On your bedside table

Once you've experienced hypoglycemia, make note of your symptoms and share them with your family, friends, and coworkers so they can recognize it if it happens again. When your blood glucose goes too low, your thinking and coordination may be impaired, and in extreme cases, you can lose consciousness. It's important that family, friends, and coworkers know that you have diabetes, know the signs of hypoglycemia, and know what they should do for you if you can't help yourself. If you are regularly experiencing low blood glucose, contact your diabetes care provider immediately. You probably need to have your medications adjusted.

What Can You Do to Prevent Hypoglycemia?

There are three variables that play a role in preventing hypoglycemia: medications, food, and exercise. Each influences the other in keeping your blood glucose at a safe level.

- As we explained earlier, some diabetes medications are known to contribute to hypoglycemia and some are not. Make sure you know the type of medication you take, when to take it, and whether it can cause hypoglycemia.
- Skipping meals, eating off schedule with your medication times, and not eating enough at a meal can all contribute to hypoglycemia.
- Exercise can contribute to hypoglycemia if you do not adjust the amount of food you eat or medicine you take. Pattern management can help you predict how different kinds of exercise will affect you. The intensity of the exercise and the length of time you exercise make a difference.

A Note about Exercise and Hypoglycemia

People who take insulin or another diabetes medication that can cause hypoglycemia may want to take extra precautions before exercising, especially if they are planning to do strenuous exercise or be active for more than 30 minutes.

- Before you exercise, check your blood glucose level.
- If it is at 100 mg/dL or less, eat something containing about 15 grams of carbohydrate before starting.
- Check your blood glucose again after the activity.
- Be aware that your blood glucose is likely to go down over the next few hours after activity because the body uses more glucose during and after exercise.

Let's Review

- Who usually takes insulin? *People with type 1 diabetes; most people with type 2 diabetes over time*
- What types of medication can cause hypoglycemia? *β-Blockers, insulin*

- What are three symptoms of hypoglycemia? *Pounding heart, dizziness, disorientation*
- What should you do if you are experiencing symptoms of hypoglycemia? *Check your blood glucose*

Let's Practice

Use your new knowledge and skills to work through these exercises.

- What type of diabetes medication do you take, if any? Find it in Table 10.1 or 10.2. What is its drug class? Can it cause hypoglycemia?
- Have you experienced hypoglycemia? If so, what symptoms did you experience? How did you treat it? If you haven't already, come up with a hypoglycemia plan. Here are some things to consider:
  - Who do I spend the most time with? Do they know the signs of hypoglycemia? Do they know what to do if it happens? Do they know where to find my glucose tablets or gel?
  - Do I have glucose tablets or gel on hand?
  - Where do I spend the most time (the office, the car, home)? Do I have glucose tablets or gel in all those places?

Basal/Bolus Insulin Therapy

In this chapter, you'll learn:

- Whether you're ready to move on to basal/bolus insulin therapy
- How to calculate and use your insulin-to-carbohydrate ratio
- How to calculate and use correction factors

At this point, you've learned a lot about using basic carb counting to manage your blood glucose. And if you don't use insulin, you've learned all you need to manage your blood glucose with carb counting.

But if you *do* take insulin, you may want or need to move on to basal/bolus insulin therapy. This approach is used by people who use an insulin pump or take rapid-acting insulin at mealtimes along with a once-daily dose of longer-acting insulin. If you are in one of these situations, basal/bolus therapy may help you gain some flexibility in your eating plan and better understand how to manage your blood glucose.

With basal/bolus insulin therapy, you adjust your premeal rapid-acting insulin dose to match up with the amount of carbohydrate you're going to eat in the meal. This approach gives you greater flexibility in your eating plan. However, it does involve more complex tracking and calculations than basic carb counting. The self-assessment on page 100 highlights some factors you may want to consider when deciding if basal/bolus insulin therapy is right for you.

Basal/bolus insulin therapy is used by people who use an insulin pump or take rapid-acting insulin at mealtimes along with a daily dose of longer-acting insulin.

Basal/Bolus Insulin Therapy Self-Assessment

Here are some things to consider when deciding if basal/bolus insulin therapy is right for you:

1. You use an insulin pump or take rapid-acting insulin at mealtimes.

    ☐ yes   ☐ no

2. Basic carb counting is not helping you reach your blood glucose targets.

    ☐ yes   ☐ no

3. You need more flexibility in your eating plan.

    ☐ yes   ☐ no

4. You are willing to do the math several times a day to determine your insulin dose.

    ☐ yes   ☐ no

5. You are willing and able to check your blood glucose at least four times each day.

    ☐ yes   ☐ no

6. You are willing to review your blood glucose records on a regular basis to find trends and patterns to assist in dose adjustments.

    ☐ yes   ☐ no

7. You work with a diabetes care provider, preferably a certified diabetes educator (CDE), who is willing to help you with the transition to basal/bolus insulin therapy.

    ☐ yes   ☐ no

If you can answer "yes" to most of these statements, then you may be ready to progress to basal/bolus insulin therapy.

A Note about Basal/Bolus Insulin Therapy

As explained earlier, basal/bolus insulin therapy is usually used by people who inject insulin several times a day or use an insulin pump. This approach may also be called *advanced carb counting* or *intensive diabetes management.* If you think you're ready for this approach, we encourage you to work with diabetes care providers who are knowledgeable about intensive diabetes management and are willing to give you the time you need to apply these techniques. This approach will involve regular (often weekly or more for some time) communications with your diabetes care provider over several weeks and often months to establish the most effective plan for your individual needs. **Basal/bolus insulin therapy is not a do-it-yourself approach.** This chapter will give you some basic information so you can have a more informed conversation with your diabetes care provider.

Basal/Bolus Insulin Therapy—The Ins and Outs

Here are the basics on how basal/bolus insulin therapy works:

- Before you eat, check your blood glucose.
- Figure out how much carbohydrate you'll be eating.
- Calculate how much insulin you need to "cover" the carbohydrate in your meal.
- If necessary, calculate how much insulin you need to take to bring your blood glucose into your target range.
- Take your premeal dose. This dose is the sum of the insulin to cover your carbs and any extra to bring your blood glucose into your target range.

That gives you a basic idea, but there is much more to learn about basal/bolus insulin therapy. Let's start with some vocabulary.

A New Vocabulary

As we explained above, this approach is used by people taking insulin, either from a pump or in a premeal dose. There are a lot of new terms involved with basal/bolus insulin therapy, including the language in the name itself! To use it effectively, you'll need to understand the terms on the following pages.

Basal insulin: Basal insulin is the insulin you take to help your body process the blood glucose your liver produces throughout the day. Basal insulin aims to mimic the normal insulin production of a healthy pancreas. You may also hear basal insulin referred to as "background insulin." Basal insulin needs range significantly from person to person.

An insulin pump is used to deliver a basal insulin dose, by releasing a small amount of insulin in pulses throughout the entire day. Additional basal insulin can also be delivered by injection. Newer longer-acting insulins can now deliver a basal insulin dose that lasts as long as 42 hours, making it easier than ever to maintain basal insulin levels. (See Table 10.3 in Chapter 10 to see different types of long-acting insulin and their duration times.) New insulin formulas and delivery methods are being introduced all the time; check with your diabetes care provider or CDE for the latest information.

There are many variables to consider in figuring out your basal or background insulin dose. However, don't try to figure out your background insulin dose on your own. If you require basal insulin, you will work with your diabetes care provider to determine the right basal insulin dose for you.

Bolus insulin: The amount of rapid-acting insulin you need to take before meals. This dose is a combination of your carb dose and your correction dose. The goal is for your bolus insulin dose to bring your blood glucose back to your premeal target within 3–4 hours of the start of the meal.

Total daily dose (TDD): The total amount of all types of insulin you take in 1 day. TDD is often estimated at 50% basal and 50% bolus to start, but it can vary and will change over time.

Insulin-to-carbohydrate (I:Carb or I:C) ratio: A math formula that tells you how much rapid-acting bolus insulin you need to take to cover the carbohydrate you are going to eat. For example, an I:C ratio of 1:10 means that you need 1 unit rapid-acting insulin for every 10 grams carb you eat.

Correction factor/insulin sensitivity factor (CF/ISF): A math formula that tells you how much rapid-acting bolus insulin you need to bring your blood glucose back into your target range when it is high. For example, a correction factor of 1:50 means that you need to take 1 unit of rapid-acting insulin for every 50 mg/dL your current blood glucose is over your target blood glucose. Another way to look at it: 1 unit of insulin will decrease your blood glucose by 50 mg/dL.

Target blood glucose or goal: For the purposes of basal/bolus insulin therapy, this is often estimated at 120 mg/dL. But remember, blood glucose targets vary from person to person. Your diabetes care team will work with you to set targets that are right for you.

Postprandial blood glucose (PPG): Your blood glucose level 1–2 hours after you eat. (*Post* means "after"; *prandial* means "relating to a meal.") The American Diabetes Association target for PPG is 180 mg/dL or less. This target is a critical checkpoint for people using basal/bolus insulin therapy. It is the way to see how well your bolus doses and I:C ratios are working.

Multiple daily injection (MDI) regimen: Another name for the practice of injecting basal and bolus insulin several times a day.

Insulin action time: The amount of time it takes for insulin to start working in your body. Different types of insulin have different insulin action times. You will see three different types of insulin action times: *onset*, or when it starts working; *peak*, or when it reaches its maximum effect; and *duration*, or how long it remains active.

Managing Insulin Action

Now that you're familiar with some of the terminology, let's talk some more about how basal/bolus insulin therapy works. This approach depends on you being able to manage your blood glucose proactively. In other words, you predict what your body is going to need and deliver it ahead of time.

As we explained in Chapter 10, rapid- or fast-acting insulin affects your blood glucose for 3–4 hours after you take it. So, your dose depends on what you think your body will do in the future. You can learn to predict that based on what you eat or plan to eat, what you do, and all of the other factors we've discussed that can affect blood glucose.

More about the I:C Ratio

In the vocabulary section above, we defined I:C ratio as a math formula that tells you how much rapid-acting bolus insulin you need to take to cover the carbohydrate you are going to eat. Just as with blood glucose targets, I:C ratios vary from person to person. The I:C ratio is not something you should try to figure out on your own—you'll work with your diabetes care provider to determine a starting point. We'll explain a little more here to help you have a more informed discussion with your diabetes care provider, but talk to your providers before trying to use an I:C ratio in your care plan.

The I:C ratio is not something you should try to figure out on your own—you'll work with your diabetes care provider to determine a starting point.

The first number in the I:C ratio represents the number of units of insulin you need to take. The second number represents the grams of carbohydrate you plan to eat. So, an I:C ratio of 1:10 means that you need to take 1 unit of insulin for every 10 grams of carbohydrate in the meal.

People who are sensitive to insulin—meaning that small amounts of insulin lower their blood glucose rapidly—might need a higher I:C ratio, such as 1:20. Conversely, people who are resistant to insulin—meaning it takes a lot of insulin to lower their blood glucose—might need a lower I:C ratio, such as 1:5. To make things even more interesting, you might find that you need to use different I:C ratios at different times of the day. For example, some people who eat the same amount of carbohydrate at breakfast, lunch, and dinner need more insulin in the morning than they do at lunch or dinner.

Using Your Records to Determine Your I:C Ratio

Usually, your food diary and blood glucose records are the first places your diabetes care provider will look when determining your ideal I:C ratio. In most cases, your CDE will ask you to keep detailed records for 2 weeks, recording the following information:

- All insulin doses (basal and bolus) and the times you took them
- All meals, drinks, and snacks; the times you consumed them; and the amount of carb in each of them
- All blood glucose readings and the times you took them (you may be asked to check your blood glucose more frequently than usual during the 2-week recording period)

Your diabetes care provider will then use all that data to figure out how your body reacts to food and insulin at different times of the day.

The Guideline of 500

The Guideline of 500 is another method used to calculate an I:C ratio. It uses a set number to represent the total grams of carbohydrate eaten in a day. It is called "the guideline of 500" because many clinicians use 500 as that number, especially for people who take rapid-acting insulin. (Some recommend using 450 instead, particularly for people who take regular insulin. If you need to move to this method, your diabetes care provider will tell you the number to use for the calculation.) Whatever number you use, you'll divide it by your total daily dose (TDD) of insulin (defined above). The resulting number becomes the second number in your I:C ratio.

Let's look at an example. Say your TDD is 42 units. Using the guideline of 500, you'd divide 500 by 42.

$$500 \div 42 = 12$$

This equation estimates an I:C ratio of 1:12, or 1 unit of rapid-acting insulin for every 12 grams of carbohydrate you eat in a meal or snack.

If your I:C ratio is 1:12, and you eat a breakfast with 60 grams of carbohydrate in it, how much insulin are you going to take to cover the carbohydrate in the meal? Divide the total carbohydrate in the meal by the second number in your I:C ratio:

$$60 \text{ grams} \div 12 = 5$$

So you will take 5 units of insulin to cover the 60 grams of carbohydrate in the meal.

You can see that you get two different results from the food log method and the guideline of 500. This is why it is so important to work with a CDE when using carb counting for basal/bolus insulin therapy. There are many factors that influence your basal and bolus insulin doses, and they can vary greatly from person to person. A CDE can help you figure this out and find what works best for you.

What if Your Blood Glucose Is High *Before* You Eat?

You've learned that your premeal insulin dose should bring your blood glucose back to your premeal target within 3–4 hours of the start of the meal. But what if your blood glucose level is above your premeal target *before* you even start eating? When this happens, you may need some additional insulin to get your blood glucose on target. This is called a "correction factor" or "correction dose."

How to Determine Your Glucose Correction Factor

There are two steps to calculating your correction factor. First, use the 1800 Rule. That means dividing 1,800 by your TDD. So, if your TDD is 35, it would look like this:

$$1{,}800 \div 35 = 51 \text{ (round down to 50)}$$

This equation estimates a correction factor of 1:50, meaning that 1 unit of rapid-acting insulin lowers your blood glucose by 50 mg/dL. (If you take short-acting insulin, your diabetes care provider may recommend using the number 1,500 instead of 1,800 for better accuracy.)

Once you have your correction factor, you can use it to determine a correction insulin dose. Let's say you check your blood glucose before dinner, and it is 210 mg/dL. Your target premeal blood glucose level is 110 mg/dL. To find out how much you need to lower your blood glucose to get to your target, you subtract the target blood glucose from the actual blood glucose number on your meter.

210 (actual blood glucose)
−   110 (target level)

_____

100 (the difference between where you are and where you want to be)

Now you use your correction factor to figure out how many units of insulin you need to lower your blood glucose by 100 mg/dL. If your correction factor is 1:50, you'd do the following calculation:

$$100 \div 50 = 2 \text{ units of insulin}$$

So, you need to take 2 units of insulin to get your blood glucose to your target level. (If you arrive at a number with a fraction and use a device that counts in whole numbers, you can round down. If you use a pump, you can take the exact dose.)

Using the Correction Factor to Figure Your Insulin Dose

Now you know your correction dose, and you know your regular dose based on your I:C factor. Now you need to add them together to determine your total premeal insulin dose. Using the amounts in the previous examples, we know that you need 5 units of insulin to cover the 60 grams of carbohydrate in your breakfast, *and* you need 2 units of insulin to bring your blood glucose back to your premeal target. So, to figure how much rapid-acting insulin to take, you add the two results together:

$$\begin{array}{r} 5 \text{ units for the meal} \\ + \quad 2 \text{ units to correct premeal levels} \\ \hline 7 \text{ units of insulin} \end{array}$$

Write It Down

Keep track of your current correction factor and I:C ratio and carry it with you. Keep it on a slip of paper in your wallet or in a note on your smartphone. This way, if you forget, you know where to look. Be sure to update it when your correction factor and I:C ratios change.

....

What if Your Blood Glucose Is Too Low Before You Eat?

If your blood glucose is too low before a meal (<70 mg/dL), treat the low first. Follow the Rule of 15 reviewed in Chapter 10: eat something with about 15 grams of carbohydrate, wait 15 minutes, and check your blood glucose again. Once your glucose is back in your target range, use your I:C ratio as usual to figure out your mealtime dose.

What if These Formulas Aren't Working for Me?

If you find that these formulas aren't helping you arrive at the best insulin dose and your blood glucose levels are not on target, talk to your diabetes care provider or CDE. They can work with you to fine-tune your basal/bolus insulin therapy. This approach is a process and will require continual review of your food logs, blood glucose records, and insulin doses to help you keep your blood glucose in your target range.

....

When to Take Mealtime Insulin

As a general rule, it's best to take your premeal insulin dose about 15 minutes before you start eating when you can. But of course, this is not always possible in real life.

If you're in a situation where you're not sure how much you're going to eat, or how much carb it contains, take your best guess and calculate a starting dose. If you eat more, you can always take another small dose of insulin to cover the additional grams of carb.

If you use an insulin pump, you can do this with a split dose or extended dose. Here's how it works: 15 minutes before you eat, you tell your pump to deliver an insulin dose up front that will cover the amount of carbs that you're sure you are going to eat. Then you tell your pump to deliver the rest of the dose gradually over the next 30–60 minutes. This technique works especially well if you're eating a large meal, because larger-than-normal meals can cause slower rises in blood glucose levels. This process is also helpful if you're eating a longer meal, like at a lengthy dinner party. In situations like these, it may be better to test your blood glucose before eating the rest of the meal to help you calculate your insulin dose. As you can see, using split or extended doses can be tricky; talk with your CDE about how to calculate and program your pump for split or extended doses.

What if you're at a restaurant and your food takes a long time to come out? If you are unsure when your food will arrive, to be safe, wait and take your dose when it arrives.

Be Careful about "Stacking" Insulin

Sometimes, you may be tempted to take more insulin while your last dose is still in your bloodstream. Perhaps your blood glucose hasn't come down as far as you expected, and you think a little more insulin will help you reach your target.

This is called "stacking insulin," and it can be dangerous. **You should not use a correction dose until after your insulin's duration of action period is over.** As a general rule, don't take a correction dose within 4 hours of your last insulin dose.

Let's look at an example to make the concept clearer. Let's say you take a premeal dose of rapid-acting insulin before lunch. Three hours later, you have a snack with 35 grams of carbohydrate. When you check your blood glucose as you're eating the snack, it is 195 mg/dL. You want to get your blood glucose down to your premeal target of 120 mg/dL, so you calculate that you need 2 units of insulin (your correction dose), and another 2 units to cover the carbohydrate in the snack. You take 4 units of insulin, and several hours later, your blood glucose is 55 mg/dL. Why?

In this example, your blood glucose is dangerously low because you didn't consider that there was still at least one hour of action left in your pre-lunch rapid-acting insulin dose. People who use insulin pumps sometimes call this "insulin on board." Whatever you call it, it can be dangerous.

Because of this danger, different types of insulin specify their duration of action (see Table 10.3 in Chapter 10). The duration of action is usually listed as a range, such as 3–5 hours, because the duration of action can vary from person to person. Remember, insulin stays active in your bloodstream for about 2 hours *after* its peak. Be patient, and you're likely to see your glucose back down to target levels before your next meal.

Over time, you'll learn how long your doses stay in your system, based on the dose, the time of day, and your activity level around that time. While you're learning, it's important to keep careful records and check your blood glucose levels frequently so you can get a sense of how your body reacts to your insulin dose.

As you can imagine, disregarding "stacked insulin" is a common cause of hypoglycemia. Talk to your diabetes care provider about how to avoid this situation. He or she may suggest using a higher premeal blood glucose target for your calculation when you're taking additional insulin before the previous dose is cleared from your system. If you use an insulin pump, be aware that many pumps have a built-in feature that helps you consider your previous bolus dose before initiating your next dose.

We hope that this chapter has helped you become more comfortable with basal/bolus insulin therapy. But remember, this is an ongoing process. Even after lots of practice, there will be times that your I:C ratio is not quite right and your blood glucose is higher than your target ranges. When this happens, go back to the basics. Measure your serving sizes and the amount of carbohydrate in them. See if your portions have grown or shrunk. Review your label reading and interpretation skills and check those for accuracy. Go through your checklist of things in your life that could have changed—your weight, your activity level, your medications. Doing these quick "quality assurance" checks every so often is helpful. Intensive diabetes management requires an ongoing daily commitment. But over time, these techniques will become second nature. Remember, this is all in the name of your health—feeling your best right now, and far into the future.

Let's Review

See if you can answer these questions. Refer back to the chapter if you need help.

- Who is basal/bolus insulin therapy for? *People who inject insulin several times a day or use an insulin pump*

- What is an I:C ratio? *A math formula that tells you how much rapid-acting bolus insulin you need to take to cover the carbohydrate you are going to eat*
- What is TDD? *Total daily dose. The total amount of insulin taken in one day*
- What is a correction factor? *A math formula that tells you how much rapid-acting bolus insulin you need to bring your blood glucose back into your target range when it is high*
- What is stacked insulin? *When you take another insulin dose before the action time of the previous dose has ended*

Let's Practice

Work through the following examples to practice your skills.

- Your I:C ratio is 1:15, your ISF is 1:50, and your blood glucose is 165 mg/dL. How much insulin should you take before eating a meal with 50 grams of carbohydrate?
- Your TDD is 30. How would you figure out your correction factor?
- Figure out an insulin dose using the following information:
  - Premeal blood glucose is 175 mg/dL
  - Target premeal blood glucose is 120 mg/dL
  - Correction factor is 1 unit to lower blood glucose 70 mg/dL
  - Amount of carbohydrate in the meal is 69 grams
  - I:C ratio is 1:16

Appendix (1)

Carb Counts of Everyday Foods

There are a variety of convenient online resources for finding the carb count of foods we eat. Appendix 2 includes a list of websites and smartphone apps you can explore. In this appendix, we've listed information on many common foods to provide an easy reference while you work through the book. As a general rule, it is better to get your information from the Nutrition Facts label, but this handy list can help when you don't have a label available. These numbers are estimates; actual nutrient content can vary.

Starches

Starches include breads, cereals, grains, crackers, snacks, beans, peas, lentils, and starchy foods prepared with fat. Some vegetables, like potatoes and corn, are considered "starchy" as well; see Vegetables below.

Starches	Serving	Calories	Carb (g)
BREADS			
Bagel	1 large	312	60
Bread, pumpernickel	1 slice	80	15
Bread, raisin	1 slice	71	14
Bread, rye	1 slice	83	16
Bread, white, reduced-calorie	1 slice	48	10
Bread, white	1 slice	67	12
Bread, whole-wheat	1 slice	69	13
English muffin	1 muffin	134	26
Hamburger bun or roll	1	120	22
Hot dog bun	1	122	22
Pita bread (6" diameter)	1	164	34
Roll, plain dinner	1 oz	85	14
Tortilla, corn, 6–7"	1	52	11
Tortilla, flour, 6"	1	112	15
Waffle, toaster-style, 4" square	1	96	15
CEREALS			
All-Bran	1/2 cup	81	23
Cheerios	1/2 cup	50	10
Cornflakes	1/2 cup	50	12
Cream of rice	1/2 cup	314	71
Cream of wheat	1 packet	150	30
Fiber One Bran Cereal	1/2 cup	60	25
Granola	1/4 cup	125	19

Starches	Serving	Calories	Carb (g)
Granola cereal, low-fat	1/4 cup	86	18
Grits	1/2 cup	71	16
Oatmeal, cooked	1/2 cup	73	13
Product 19	1/2 cup	50	13
Puffed rice	1/2 cup	26	6
Puffed wheat	1/2 cup	22	5
Raisin bran	1/2 cup	95	23
Rice Krispies	1/2 cup	52	12
Shredded wheat, plain	1/2 cup	83	20
Wheaties	1/2 cup	67	15

CRACKERS AND SNACKS

	Serving	Calories	Carb (g)
Animal crackers	8	89	15
Crispbread	2 slices	73	16
Graham crackers	3	99	18
Matzos	1 cracker	111	23
Melba toast	4 slices	78	15
Oyster crackers	20	86	14
Pita chips, baked	10 chips	130	19
Popcorn, microwave, 94% fat-free	3 cups	65	14
Popcorn, microwave, with butter	3 cups	96	11
Popcorn, popped, no salt or fat added	3 cups	93	19
Potato chips	15 chips	160	15
Potato chips, baked	15 chips	120	23
Pretzels, sticks	15 pretzels	100	23
Rice cakes, plain	2	70	15
Tortilla chips	11 chips	150	17
Tortilla chips, baked	14 chips	120	22

(continued on next page)

Starches	Serving	Calories	Carb (g)
GRAINS			
Bulgur, cooked	1/2 cup	76	17
Cornmeal, dry, yellow	3 Tbsp	83	18
Couscous, cooked	1/2 cup	88	18
Flour, white	3 Tbsp	85	18
Kasha, cooked	1/2 cup	100	20
Millet, cooked	1/2 cup	104	20
Rice, white, long-grain, cooked	1/2 cup	103	22
Rice, brown, cooked	1/2 cup	109	23
Wheat germ, toasted	3 Tbsp	81	11
PASTA			
Macaroni, elbows, cooked	1/2 cup	111	22
Noodles, enriched egg, cooked	1/2 cup	110	20
Spaghetti, cooked	1/2 cup	91	18
BEANS, PEAS, AND LENTILS			
Beans, baked	1/2 cup	140	29
Beans, kidney, canned	1/2 cup	105	19
Beans, kidney, cooked	1/2 cup	112	20
Beans, lima, canned, drained	1/2 cup	99	18
Beans, lima, frozen, cooked	1/2 cup	76	14
Beans, navy, cooked	1/2 cup	129	24
Beans, pinto, cooked	1/2 cup	122	22
Beans, white, cooked	1/2 cup	125	23
Chickpeas, cooked	1/2 cup	134	23
Lentils, cooked	1/2 cup	115	20
Peas, split, cooked	1/2 cup	116	21
Peas, black-eyed, cooked	1/2 cup	100	17

Vegetables

This chart includes raw, fresh, and canned vegetables and vegetable juices.

Vegetables	Serving	Calories	Carb (g)
NONSTARCHY			
Artichoke, cooked	1 medium	53	12
Artichoke hearts, canned, drained	4 pieces	25	1
Asparagus, frozen, cooked	1 cup	32	3.5
Bean sprouts, canned	1/2 cup	12	1.5
Beans, green, fresh, cooked	1/2 cup	22	5
Beets, canned, drained	1/2 cup	40	8
Broccoli, fresh, cooked	1/2 cup	27	5.5
Brussels sprouts, frozen, cooked	1/2 cup	33	6.5
Cabbage, fresh, shredded	1/2 cup	17	4
Carrots, cooked	1/2 cup	27	6
Carrots, fresh, raw	1 cup	52	5
Cauliflower, fresh, raw	1 cup	27	5
Celery, fresh, raw	1 cup	17	4
Chard, Swiss, cooked	1/2 cup	18	4
Collard greens, fresh, cooked	1/2 cup	26	6
Cucumber, raw	1 cup	16	4
Eggplant, fresh, cooked	1/2 cup	17	4
Endive/escarole, raw	1 cup	9	2
Green (spring) onions	1 cup	32	7
Kale, raw, chopped	1/2 cup	18	4
Leeks, fresh, cooked	1/2 cup	16	4
Mushrooms, fresh, raw	1 cup	15	2
Mustard greens, fresh, cooked	1/2 cup	10	2
Okra, frozen, cooked	1/2 cup	34	5

(continued on next page)

Vegetables	Serving	Calories	Carb (g)
Onions, fresh	1 cup	67	16
Onions, fresh, cooked	1/2 cup	46	11
Pea pods (snow peas), fresh, cooked	1/2 cup	34	6
Peas, sugar snap, frozen, uncooked	1/2 cup	30	5
Pepper, green bell, raw, slices	1 cup	18	4
Pepper, red bell, fresh, cooked	1/2 cup	19	5
Pepper, hot chili, green, canned	1/2 cup	25	3
Radishes, sliced	1 cup	20	4
Spinach, fresh	1 cup	7	1
Squash, summer, fresh, cooked	1/2 cup	18	4
Squash, summer, raw	1 cup	18	4
Tomatoes, canned, regular	1/2 cup	24	6
Tomatoes, raw	1 cup	32	7
Turnip greens, fresh, cooked	1/2 cup	14	3
Turnips, cooked, cubed	1/2 cup	17	4
Water chestnuts, canned, drained	1/2 cup	40	9
Zucchini, fresh, cooked	1/2 cup, slices	14	4
Zucchini, raw	1 cup	18	4
STARCHY			
Corn, canned, drained	1/2 cup	66	15
Corn on cob, cooked	1/2 large ear	66	16
Peas, green, canned, drained, no salt added	1 cup	39	8
Peas, green, frozen, cooked	1/2 cup	62	11
Plantain, ripe, cooked	1/2 cup, slices	89	24
Potato, baked with skin	5 oz, small	134	30
Potato, white, peeled, boiled	4.4 oz, small	108	25
Squash, acorn, cubed cooked	1 cup	115	30
Yams, cooked	1/2 cup	113	27

Fruit

Fruit includes fresh, dried, canned, and frozen fruit. Fruit juices are under non-alcoholic beverages.

Fruit	Serving	Calories	Carb (g)
FRESH FRUIT			
Apple, with peel, small	1 (4 oz)	54	14
Apricots	4	67	16
Banana, small	1 (6")	72	19
Blackberries	1/2 cup	31	7
Blueberries	1/2 cup	42	11
Cantaloupe	1 cup	56	13
Cherries, sweet	12 (3 oz)	59	14
Figs, medium	2	74	19
Grapefruit	1/2	53	13
Grapes, seedless	17	60	15
Honeydew melon	1 cup	61	16
Kiwi	1	56	13
Mango	1/2 small	68	18
Nectarine	1 small	60	14
Orange	1 (6 1/2 oz)	62	15
Papaya	1 cup	55	14
Peach, medium	1 (6 oz)	57	14
Pear, large	1/2 (4 oz)	61	16
Pineapple, chunks	1 cup	83	22
Plums, small	2 (5 oz)	61	15
Raspberries, black, red	1 cup	60	14
Strawberries, halves	1 cup	49	12
Tangerine, small	2 (8 oz)	81	20
Watermelon, diced	1 cup	46	11

(continued on next page)

Fruit	Serving	Calories	Carb (g)
FRUIT, CANNED OR JARRED, WITH SOME JUICE			
Applesauce, unsweetened	1/2 cup	52	14
Apricots, juice pack	1/2 cup	59	15
Cherries, sweet, juice pack	1/2 cup	68	17
Fruit cocktail, juice pack	1/2 cup	60	14
Grapefruit sections, with juice	1 cup	74	19
Mandarin oranges, juice pack	1 cup	92	24
Peaches, juice pack	1/2 cup	55	14
Pears, juice pack	1/2 cup	62	16
Pineapple, juice pack	1/2 cup	74	20
Plums, juice pack	1/2 cup	73	19
FRUIT, DRIED			
Apples, rings	4	63	17
Apricots, halves	8	67	18
Dates	3	69	19
Figs	1 fig, small	30	8
Raisins, dark, seedless	2 Tbsp	54	14

Milk and Yogurt

Milk and yogurt includes dairy-like foods.

Milks and milk products	Serving	Calories	Carb (g)
NONFAT OR LOW-FAT			
Acidophilus milk, fat-free	1 cup	128	11
Buttermilk, fat-free	1 cup	98	12
Buttermilk, low-fat	1 cup	99	12
Lactaid, fat-free	1 cup	80	13

Milks and Milk Products	Serving	Calories	Carb (g)
Milk, 1%	1 cup	110	13
Milk, 2%	1 cup	130	12
Milk, evaporated, fat-free	1/2 cup	100	15
Milk, fat-free	1 cup	90	13
Yogurt, fruit-flavored, fat-free, no added sugar	6-oz container	50	3
Yogurt, nonfat, plain	1/2 cup	60	8.5
Yogurt, plain, low-fat	1/2 cup	77	9
Yogurt, Greek, plain, low-fat	1/2 cup	85	4.5
WHOLE MILKS			
Milk, evaporated, whole	1/2 cup	169	13
Milk, goat, whole	1 cup	168	11
Milk, whole	1 cup	150	12
Yogurt, plain, made from whole milk	1 cup	160	12
DAIRY-LIKE FOODS			
Rice drink, fat-free or 1%, plain	1 cup	90	18
Rice drink, low-fat, flavored	1 cup	122	25
Soy milk, light	1 cup	100	15
Soy milk, regular, plain	1 cup	115	11

Meat and Other Foods That Contain Mostly Protein and Fat

Most meats (such as beef, poultry, seafood, and eggs) contain no carbohydrate. However, some foods in this food group—processed meats, tofu, cheeses, and peanut butter—contain very small amounts of carbohydrate. Note the fat content in this table below. As we discussed in Chapter 6, high-fat meats can affect the way your blood glucose reacts to a meal.

Proteins	Serving	Calories	Carb (g)	Fat (g)
Beef, jerky, dried	1 oz	116	3	7
Beef sticks, smoked	1 oz	156	2	14
Cheese, American, fat-free	1 slice	31	3	0
Cheese, American, regular	1 slice	79	0	7
Cheese, cheddar, regular	1 slice	113	0	9
Cheese, Monterey jack, regular	1 slice	110	0	9
Cheese, Swiss, regular	1 slice	106	2	8
Cottage cheese, low-fat (1%)	1/2 cup	81	3	1
Cottage cheese, fat-free	1/2 cup	90	8	0
Fish sticks	2	139	12	7
Peanut butter, chunky	1 Tbsp	94	4	8
Peanut butter, smooth	1 Tbsp	94	3	8
Ricotta, part-skim	1/4 cup	86	3	5
Tempeh	1/4 cup	80	4	5
Tofu	1/2 cup	183	5	11

Sweets and Sugary Foods

The grams of carbohydrate per serving in this group vary quite a bit. The calorie content varies quite a bit, too.

Sweets	Serving	Calories	Carb (g)
Angel food cake, not frosted	1 slice (2 oz)	128	29
Brownie, unfrosted	2" square	115	18
Cake, frosted	2" square	175	29
Cake, unfrosted	2" square	97	17
Cookies, chocolate chip	2 medium	156	19
Cookies, gingersnap, regular	3	87	16
Cookies, sandwich, cream filling	2 small	93	14
Cookies, sugar-free	3 small	141	20
Cookies, vanilla wafers	5	88	15
Cupcake, plain	1	200	23
Danish pastry, fruit type (4 1/4" diameter)	1 pastry	263	34
Donut, glazed (3 3/4" diameter)	1	239	30
Donut, plain cake	1 medium	196	21
Fruit spreads, 100% fruit	1 Tbsp	40	11
Granola bar	1	134	18
Granola bar, chewy, low-fat	1	109	22
Honey	1 Tbsp	64	17
Ice cream	1/2 cup	165	15
Ice cream, fat-free	1/2 cup	90	22
Ice cream, light	1/2 cup	120	16
Ice cream, no sugar added	1/2 cup	115	15
Jam or preserves, regular	1 Tbsp	48	13
Jelly, regular	1 Tbsp	52	13
Pie, fruit, 2-crust	1/6 pie	284	42

(continued on next page)

Sweets	Serving	Calories	Carb (g)
Pie, pumpkin or custard	1/8 pie	168	22
Pudding, regular, reduced-fat milk	1/2 cup	141	26
Pudding, sugar-free, fat-free, fat-free milk	1/2 cup	70	12
Sherbet	1/2 cup	138	29
Sorbet	1/2 cup	130	31
Sweet roll	1	264	36
Syrup, pancake, light	2 Tbsp	50	13
Syrup, pancake, regular	1 Tbsp	50	13
Yogurt, frozen, fat-free, no-sugar-added vanilla	1/2 cup	70	18
Yogurt, frozen, regular	1/2 cup	110	19

Fats

Many of the foods in the fat group—margarine, butter, oils—contain no carbo-hydrate. So they don't figure into carb counting. However, you'll still want to limit your intake of them because they contribute a lot of calories and fat. Several foods in this food group—nuts, salad dressings, mayonnaise, and other spreads—contain small amounts of carbohydrate.

Fats	Serving	Calories	Carb (g)	Fat (g)
NUTS				
Almonds, raw	1 oz (23 nuts)	164	6	14
Cashews, raw	1 oz (18 nuts)	157	9	12
Peanuts, raw	1 oz (28 nuts)	161	5	14
Pecan halves, raw	1 oz (10 halves)	196	4	20
Pumpkin seeds, roasted, no salt added	1 oz (150 seeds)	148	4	12
Walnut halves	1 oz (14 halves)	183	4	18

Fats	Serving	Calories	Carb (g)	Fat (g)
SALAD DRESSINGS, SPREADS, AND CONDIMENTS				
Hummus	1 Tbsp	23	2	1
Ketchup	1 Tbsp	15	4	0
Mayonnaise, regular	1 Tbsp	57	4	5
Mayonnaise, fat-free	1 Tbsp	13	3	0
Mayonnaise, reduced-fat	1 Tbsp	49	1	5
Mustard, yellow	1 Tbsp	10	1	1
Salad dressing, blue cheese	1 Tbsp	76	1	8
Salad dressing, blue cheese, fat-free	1 Tbsp	14	2	0
Salad dressing, Caesar	1 Tbsp	78	1	9
Salad dressing, Caesar, reduced-fat	1 Tbsp	17	3	1
Salad dressing, French	1 Tbsp	73	3	7
Salad dressing, French, fat-free	1 Tbsp	21	5	0
Salad dressing, French, reduced-fat	1 Tbsp	37	5	2
Salad dressing, Italian	1 Tbsp	43	2	4
Salad dressing, Italian, fat-free	1 Tbsp	7	1	0
Salad dressing, Italian, reduced-fat	1 Tbsp	11	1	1
Salad dressing, Ranch	1 Tbsp	73	1	8
Salad dressing, Ranch, fat-free	1 Tbsp	17	4	0
Salad dressing, Ranch, reduced-fat	1 Tbsp	33	2	3
Salad dressing, Thousand Island	1 Tbsp	59	3	6
Salad dressing, Thousand Island, fat-free	1 Tbsp	21	5	0
Salad dressing, Thousand Island, reduced-fat	1 Tbsp	31	3	2

Beverages: Nonalcoholic

Many drinks don't contain carbohydrate, but some do. This list covers fruit and vegetable juices and other drinks (except milk).

Beverage	Serving	Calories	Carb (g)
Apple juice/cider	8 fl oz	120	29
Caffe latte, nonfat milk	8 fl oz	67	10
Caffe latte, whole milk	8 fl oz	136	11
Caffe mocha, nonfat milk, no whipped cream	8 fl oz	112	21
Caffe mocha, 2% milk, no whipped cream	8 fl oz	136	21
Coffee, black	8 fl oz	2	0
Coffee, with 2 Tbsp half-and-half	8 fl oz	41	1
Fruit juice blends, 100% juice	8 fl oz	120	29
Grape juice	8 fl oz	170	42
Orange juice, fresh	8 fl oz	112	26
Pineapple juice, canned	8 fl oz	128	32
Prune juice	8 fl oz	180	42
Soda, cola	12 oz	131	34
Soda, cola, diet	12 oz	7	1
Soda, ginger ale	12 oz	124	32
Soda, lemon lime	12 oz	139	35
Sport drink, regular	16 oz	112	28
Sport drink, sweetened with a no-calorie sweetener	16 oz	20	4
Tomato juice	1/2 cup	21	5
Vegetable juice	1/2 cup	25	6

Beverages: Alcoholic

Most of the calories in alcoholic beverages are provided by the alcohol. Most alcoholic beverages contain no carbohydrate, but other beverages do, so consider that when you order mixed drinks. When you drink alcohol, be careful because alcohol can either make your blood glucose rise or fall too low. See Chapter 6 for more information on the use of alcoholic beverages. Note that these are average figures. Different products may have different nutritional value.

Alcoholic beverage	Serving	Calories	Carb (g)
Beer, regular	12 oz	153	13
Beer, light	12 oz	103	5
Liquor, any type (e.g., gin, rum, vodka)	1 1/2 oz (1 shot)	97	0
Liqueur, any type (e.g., Kahlua, crème de menthe)	1 1/2 oz (1 shot)	175	24
Wine, red	5 oz	126	4
Wine, white	5 oz	121	4

For more information about carb counts of everyday foods, see *Choose Your Foods: Food Lists for Diabetes*, a booklet from the Academy of Nutrition and Dietetics and American Diabetes Association.

Appendix (2)

Carb Counting Resources

These days, you can find tons of information and resources on just about anything via the Internet. The same is true for diabetes and carb counting! Enter either term into any search engine, and you'll receive pages of lists. That being said, it can be hard to tell which sites provide accurate, scientifically based, unbiased information. Below are a few questions to ask yourself, provided by the National Institutes of Health (NIH).

Checking Out Online Sources of Health Information: Five Quick Questions

If you're visiting an online health site for the first time or downloading a new app, ask these five questions:

1. **Who** runs or created the site or app? Can you trust them?
2. **What** is the site or app promising or offering? Do its claims seem too good to be true?
3. **When** was its information written or reviewed? Is it up-to-date?
4. **Where** does the information come from? Is it based on scientific research?
5. **Why** does the site or app exist? Is it selling something?

It's also always a good idea to run new information, products, or sources by your diabetes care team. You can ask them for recommendations, too. They'll be happy to share their favorite books, websites, apps, and tools. Here are some of our favorites.

Books

Check out the selection at your local library, so you can review books before investing in your own copies. The American Diabetes Association retail site, www.shopdiabetes.org, has a whole section devoted to books. And of course, you can find just about anything on Amazon.com. Some publications are available in e-book versions, too. Here are some favorites that relate specifically to carb counting.

- *The Diabetes Carbohydrate and Fat Gram Guide*, by Lea Ann Holzmeister, RD, CDE (American Diabetes Association, 5th edition, 2017). This book provides the carbohydrate count, as well as other nutrition information, for thousands of foods, including fruits, vegetables, and other produce; meats, poultry, and seafood; desserts; many foods you know by brand name; frozen entrées; and more. Available on www.shopdiabetes.org.
- *The CalorieKing Calorie, Fat & Carbohydrate Counter*, by Allan Borushek (Family Health Publications, 2018). This book provides the calorie, fat, and carbohydrate information for thousands of basic and brand-name foods. Available at www.calorieking.com/products/books/.
- *Eat Out, Eat Well*, by Hope Warshaw, MMSc, RD, CDE (American Diabetes Association, 2015). This easy-to-carry guide provides practical and realistic solutions to eating healthier when eating out in nearly every type of restaurant—from fast food to fine dining—and nearly every cuisine—from Italian and Mexican to Indian and Japanese. Available at www.shopdiabetes.org.
- *Nutrition in the Fast Lane—The Fast Food Dining Guide* (20th edition, 2017). This booklet, updated annually, provides the nutrition information for 54 of the country's most popular chain restaurants. Available at www.fastfoodfacts.com or by calling 800-634-1993.

Websites

- www.diabetes.org
  The website of the American Diabetes Association. Provides a wealth of information on everything from self-management to medications to recipes. This

website also includes tools to help you locate diabetes care providers and support groups in your area.

- www.diabeteseducator.org
The website of the American Association of Diabetes Educators. This website is designed primarily for certified diabetes educators (CDEs), but its Living with Diabetes section includes excellent resources for the layperson. You can also use the site to help you find a CDE in your area or to find group classes you can join.

- www.nutrition.gov
This is a U.S. Department of Agriculture (USDA)–sponsored website that offers credible information to help you make healthful eating choices. This link will take you to the home page; scroll down to click on the link for the USDA Food Composition Databases, which provides complete nutritional information on over 8,000 foods. You can change the serving size and the site will recalculate all the nutrient data for you.

- www.choosemyplate.gov
This is another USDA website targeted at consumers. It provides information on planning healthy meals, physical activity, and portion control.

- www.healthydiningfinder.com
This website allows you to search for restaurants that offer a selection of healthier menu items and view the nutrition information for those items. You can search by zip code and/or other criteria. The site was developed with a grant from the Centers for Disease Control and Prevention (CDC) and in collaboration with the National Restaurant Association. New restaurants are added regularly.

- www.calorieking.com
A comprehensive nutritional database the provides nutrient breakdown of thousands of foods. A smartphone app is also available to allow you to search the database on the go.

- www.myfooddiary.com
This site provides a food database, food diary, exercise tracker, nutritional analysis, and more. It offers a free 7-day trial; after that, you pay $9 per month for access.

- www.nutritiondata.com
This website, sponsored by *Self* magazine, is free and offers a ton of great features. There's a food diary, an exercise tracker, and functionality to help

you analyze the nutrient content of recipes. You can store favorite recipes and favorite foods, and set specific nutrient goals (like carbs!) to help you stay on track.

- **www.dlife.com**
  DLife says its goal is to "address the overwhelming need for real, practical solutions to the 24/7 challenge of managing diabetes." It offers a wealth of resources, from a "Diabetes 101" educational section to news of new diabetes research to information on carb counting, recipes, and more.

- **www.diabetesnet.com**
  DiabetesNet calls itself "the diabetes mall." It offers all sorts of diabetes information, from patient education to food logs to research to device information. It also includes links to other helpful resources and sites.

Smartphone/Tablet Apps

New smartphone apps are coming out all the time. Enter "diabetes" in the search field on your phone's App Store or Google Play, and you'll see dozens. Beware—with the popularity of low-carb diets, you're likely to see many "carb counting" apps for weight loss. (If they reference Atkins or Keto, they're designed for low-carb diets, not diabetic carb counting.) Some apps are free, and some have a small cost associated with them (anywhere from 99 cents to $5). Others offer a free version with basic functionality, with the option to upgrade to a paid version later. All apps have websites also (listed below), so visit a few to compare features. It's always a good idea to start with the free version if that option exists, to see how you like the app before paying for extras. If you use a blood glucose meter or an insulin pump, the manufacturers may offer a free app as well.

- **MyMacros** (https://getmymacros.com) Available in the App Store (Apple) and Google Play (Android). One-time charge of $2.99. Includes a food database and ability to set daily and mealtime goals for various macronutrients (which includes carbs). You can also add custom foods for things you don't find in the database.

- **MyFitnessPal** (www.myfitnesspal.com) Available in the App Store (Apple) and Google Play (Android). Free. Incudes a food database, customizable food plans, and discussion forums. Can also be synced with other apps and devices, like Fitbit Tracker and MapMyRun.

- Glucose Buddy (www.glucosebuddy.com) Available in the App Store (Apple) and Google Play (Android). Free version with basic functionality, premium version $59.99 per year. Allows you to track blood glucose meter readings and graph them to easily spot trends.
- MySugr (www.mysugr.com) Available in the App Store (Apple) and Google Play (Android). Free version with basic functionality, Pro version costs $2.99 a month or $27.99 for a year. The free version provides access to a food database and food diary.
- SparkPeople (www.sparkpeople.com) SparkPeople is not specifically for people with diabetes—it is primarily a weight loss app. But the SparkPeople community includes many resources for people with both type 1 and type 2 diabetes, including meal-planning tips, recipes, and exercise tips.

Portion Control Products

There are a variety of products available to help you manage your portion sizes and stick to your carb counting goals. Enter "portion control products" into any Internet search engine or Amazon.com and review the options. The American Diabetes Association's retail site www.shopdiabetes.org also offers many options. From the home page, select "Accessories," then choose "Meal Planning Tools" to view all available products. There are a variety of kits that include books or pamphlets, along with divided plates with travel lids, measuring tools, and educational materials.

Index

Note: Page numbers followed by *f* refer to figures. Page numbers followed by *t* refer to tables.

total daily dose (TDD), 102, 105–106
Total Fat, 20
Total Sugars, 21–22, 28
trans fat, 20–21, 52, 54, 56
triglyceride, 56
type 1 diabetes, 2, 85–86, 88, 94
type 2 diabetes, 2, 7, 54, 76, 85–86, 88

U

USDA Food Composition Databases, 129
U.S. Department of Agriculture (USDA), 129
U.S. Food and Drug Administration (FDA),
   19–20, 22–23, 25, 27–30

V

vegetable, 3, 4*t*, 5, 39–40, 115*t*–116*t*
vegetable juice, 124*t*

vision, 82, 93
vitamin, 22, 52

W

Warshaw, Hope, Eat Out, Eat Well, 128
website, 14–15, 44, 48, 61, 67–68, 71–73, 80,
   127–130
weight loss, 6–8, 25
weights and measures, 36
whole grain, 23–24
Whole Grain Stamp, 24*f*, 25

X

xylitol, 30*t*

Y

yogurt, 118*t*–119*t*